THE
JOY DIET

.

MARTHA BECK

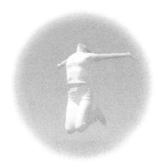

THE
JOY DIET

•

10 Daily Practices for a Happier Life

CROWN PUBLISHERS

NEW YORK

For credits, see page 227.

Copyright © 2003 by Martha Beck

Published by Crown Publishers, New York, New York.
Member of the Crown Publishing Group,
a division of Random House, Inc.
www.randomhouse.com

CROWN is a trademark and the Crown colophon is a registered trademark of Random House, Inc.

Printed in the United States of America

Design by Lynne Amft

Library of Congress Cataloging-in-Publication Data
Beck, Martha Nibley, 1962–
The joy diet ten daily practices for a happier life / Martha Beck.
1. Happiness.   2. Joy.   3. Self-realization.   I. Title.
BF575.H27B43   2003
158.1—dc21
2002154784

ISBN 0-609-60990-4

10 9

First Edition

To the Extreme Brady Bunch,
immediate and extended.
I love you all forever.

AUTHOR'S NOTE

This book uses illustrative examples I've collected during many sessions I've spent with my life-coaching clients. Though the substance of each anecdote is true, I have disguised the clients' identities by changing their names and other descriptive details. The same goes for the stories I've snitched from friends and relatives, except for my immediate family, whose names and descriptions are included with flagrant accuracy.

ACKNOWLEDGMENTS

To begin with, I'd like to acknowledge my clients, whose trust and hard work makes my job so fulfilling. I hope this book communicates some of the pride, gratitude, and love I feel as I watch them change their lives.

My heartfelt thanks to many people at Crown Publishers who helped make this book possible. Betsy Rapoport, the best editor in the history of earth, gave me the idea for *The Joy Diet,* and helped me develop many of its components. No one more brilliant, talented, and kind has ever wielded a tally-counter in one hand and a margarita in the other. The hilarious and compassionate Chip Gibson was a stalwart believer in my work before anyone else had ever heard of it. Stephanie Higgs shouldered way more than her share of work involved in getting *The Joy Diet* through the publication process, for which I will always feel gratitude and guilt. Steve Ross has championed my writing, offered heartening feedback when I needed it most, and made himself continuously available despite his many other obligations.

My agent, Beth Vesel, moves effortlessly from the role of babysitter to businessperson, and I'm eternally grateful for the work in both capacities.

I have learned so much from the wonderful staff of *O, The Oprah Magazine,* especially my editor, Mamie Healey, and the amazing Amy Gross. Their wisdom, unerring discernment, and gentle feedback have helped me grow as a writer and as a person, and I am grateful for that every day.

My deep gratitude also goes to Dr. Ruth Killpack, who put me on the path that led to *The Joy Diet,* and propped me up as I learned how to walk that path on my own. She and Dr. Rita Edmonds encouraged me to write this book when it was just a twinkle in my brain, an I am always sustained by their steadfast support.

Massive thanks to Annette Rogers, who is often my first editor and always my most enthusiastic cheering squad. I never cease to be amazed by the resilience and generosity of her friendship.

I would never have finished this book if my friend Lili hadn't kept me honest, committed, and laughing through many a forced-marched writing session. Her humor and insight permeate this book, so readers who didn't like it should definitely blame her. As for me, I owe her only love and thanks.

Finally, I'd like to thank my crazy-quilt of a family: Eggen, whose simply astonishing goodness changes my life every day; Veggie Boy, who believed in me before there was anything to believe in; Ronald Hands-On, one of the most nurturing beings I've ever met; the ever-sardonic and perceptive Kat, the wildly inspirational Add-On; and my dauntless and hilarious Lizard. Thanks, guys. Everything I know about joy, I learned from you.

MENU

INTRODUCTION

EVERY NOW AND THEN, WHEN I AM FEELING EVEN more chubby, listless, and ill than usual, I put myself on a nutritional regimen that I've cobbled together over the years. My program is gleaned from the advice of countless self-help books, magazine articles, doctors, friends, and helpful strangers. It works pretty well for me. However, it has nothing to do with this book. No, if you're looking for ways to shed that potbelly or firm your buttocks, I'm afraid you'll have to look elsewhere. As far as I'm concerned, your belly and buttocks are absolutely magnificent right now, not that I want you to send me photographs. In fact, I will never write a book about dieting in the nutritional sense, because I'm not a health or fitness expert. What I am is a life coach, and this book contains instructions for a different kind of "diet," one designed not for the body but for the soul.

When the word *diet* first entered the English language, back in 1656 when I was just a girl, it didn't refer to food intake. It meant "a way of living or thinking." A few decades later, *diet* also came to mean "a day's journey." The Joy Diet is a list of ten behaviors you can add to your way of living and thinking to enhance every day's journey through the unpredictable terrain of your existence. You can implement it gradually and watch your life become steadily more vivid and satisfying. Or you can use it as a "crash diet" in an emergency, on the day when your cat gets sick or your lover dumps you or you wake up unexpectedly transfixed by the awareness of your own mortality. The Joy Diet is simply what you can do to feel better, especially when you don't know what to do to feel better.

I subscribe to the admittedly romantic belief that each person has a "right life," a journey through this world that will bring him or her the most possible joy and fulfillment. As a life coach, my mission is to help people along the journey. My last book, *Finding Your Own North Star,* is basically a primer about how you can find your own particular right life, how you can chart your course and clear out obstacles as you move toward it, and what you can expect to encounter along the way. It's deep, transformative work that lasts a lifetime (although it most often feels like play). I consider this book both a companion volume to *North Star* and a helpful travelogue. It contains suggestions and supplies that can make your journey through life, whatever that life might be, as comfortable and happy as possible. It will remind you not to lose sight of the goal of joyful living even when the journey is grinding. These ideas are very basic, the equivalent of "Pack a lunch," "Wear sunscreen," or "Keep your matches dry." But in my work I've seen that many people never think of them, that those who do often forget, and that being reminded can make all the difference between a joyful journey and hell on wheels. Over time, I've zeroed in on a short list of ten daily practices that give my clients (to put it crudely) the most bang for their buck. The Joy Diet is that list.

Going on the Joy Diet

I once undertook the task of learning T'ai chi, the venerable martial art that is usually practiced by going through a sequence of very specific movements veeeeerrrrryyy ssssllloooowwwww-llllllyyyy, like a bear trying to dance while hibernating. I was frustrated when my teacher taught me one simple gesture (set your feet shoulder width apart, raise your arms in front of you until they're parallel to the ground), then told me I had to practice it every day for a week before I could learn the next move. Oh, give me a break, I said. I'm a quick study. Why not throw caution to the martial-arts wind and teach me *two* gestures in a week? This suggestion was politely but firmly declined. Before I can teach you any new movement, said my teacher, each gesture up to that point must feel as easy and unconscious as running your hand through your hair.

I chafed wildly at this agonizingly incremental way of learning, but I came to appreciate it deeply and apply it in many areas of my life. No matter what complex thing you're learning, from playing the piano to solving calculus equations, the trick is to break the necessary actions down into trivial-seeming behaviors, then practice these behaviors until you can do each one half-asleep, while watching television with one eye and your children with the other.

That's the method I'd like you to use when you go on the Joy Diet. I recommend that you add, *in order,* a single practice or "menu item" to your daily routine each week. In other words, begin with the first activity and do it at least once a day for seven days before adding the second activity. If, after a week, the "menu item" you're working on doesn't feel as natural and integral as breathing, take a few more days to really integrate it. You can slow down the Joy Diet as much as you like. However, you shouldn't try to speed up by trying to implement every element of the Diet at once. That doesn't allow enough time to focus on each new behavior until it becomes second nature. No matter how long it takes you, the important thing is that you continue practicing each Joy Diet behavior until going a day without doing it feels odd, like never seeing the sky. At that point, you can add another menu item.

The most difficult and time-consuming of the Joy Diet activities (see Menu Item #1) is doing nothing for a few minutes a day. The other nine items are considerably easier. If you think this means they aren't challenging, you are in for a surprise. The components of the Joy Diet create a direct connection between your conscious mind and your deep self, the part of you that knows the purpose for your life and how you are meant to achieve it. This can be terrifying. Almost all of us are used to hiding our true natures from the world at large, from our loved ones, and especially from ourselves (we do this for security, which is ironic since forgetting who we really are renders us profoundly insecure). The effect of the Joy Diet is to shine a light into our hiding places, allowing us to see and remember ourselves and our reasons for being. That can change pretty much everything in your life. I've seen jaded ex-soldiers and confident CEOs shake like freezing kittens when they contemplated some of the Joy Diet behaviors, and their fears were well-founded. Like jumping out of an airplane, the activities on the Diet are ridiculously easy, and extraordinarily difficult.

As you internalize each Joy Diet menu item, you may happen upon variations and adaptations that make the Diet more effective for you. I encourage you to follow your own experience, even if it takes you in directions I don't mention. This book is only a primer, meant to help you begin developing habits that will lead you to the most fulfilling life possible. The more you follow the Joy Diet, the more clearly your soul's voice will speak to you, and the better you'll hear the instructions for your life that only it can know. This Diet, this way of living and thinking, makes its practitioners more alike only in the unanimous pursuit of their own uniqueness. Whether you're embarking on it because of a subtle hankering for a more meaningful existence, or a life crisis that has left you stunned and bewildered, it can help you down the path toward becoming yourself. I wish you all the success in the world, and a good day's journey.

NOTHING

•

TO BEGIN THE JOY DIET, YOU MUST DO NOTHING
FOR AT LEAST FIFTEEN MINUTES A DAY.

"SOMETHING IS MISSING FROM MY LIFE."

This is the most common reason people give me for seeking my life-coaching services. Rarely do clients come to me with a clear dilemma to resolve or a simple goal to achieve. Sometimes the sense of "something missing" seems vague and inexplicable, like the phantom ache an amputee might feel in a limb that no longer exists. On other occasions, when a client is facing some kind of loss, choice, or crisis, the compulsion to find the Missing Something may be as keen and painful as glass in a wound. Often, the people who ask me to help them find the Something have traveled thousands of miles and spent substantial amounts of energy, time, and money on their search. I have nothing to offer them. Fortunately, this is exactly what they need.

Nothing, nothing at all, is the first ingredient you must add to your life when you go on the Joy Diet. Whether you're doing the program as an overall life enhancement, or using it to face some kind of trauma, I'm almost certain you need nothing—a good, strong dose of nothing, and soon. Okay, enough coy wordplay. What I mean is that the best way to break through any barrier is to access a point of perfect stillness at the center of your being, a self deeper than your senses or your mind. We modern, scientific thinkers are rarely taught that such a thing exists, much less how to connect with it. But every ancient tradition holds that from this still core of the self, this infinitely fertile emptiness, springs all that is authentic about you: your identity, your ability to recognize truth, the real operating instructions for your life.

This chapter is meant to help you recognize what you already know about the absolute peace of your own deep self; the "nothing" that will allow you to handle anything, that will teach you how to approach all your problems, from the most trivial to the most momentous. In case you have never experienced this kind of nothing, I'll first discuss it as it has been described, for millennia, by some wise beings who took the time to become intimately familiar with it. Then, since I am a thoroughgoing pragmatist, I'll give some practical instructions for adding nothing to your life—instructions that have saved my own sanity more times than I can count.

These practices can provide a sanctuary that no one can ever take from you. In the moments when your heart is tired, confused, or broken, when you have no energy to do anything, you'll naturally turn to what your true self is telling you it needs: nothing. This is always a step—usually the first step—that will move you away from suffering and toward joy.

Worshiping the Holy Something

I know all this enthusiasm about nothingness may be baffling to some of my readers, who have been socialized from the cradle to think that doing just about anything is preferable to doing nothing. Many of my clients think that a person who spends a day accomplishing nothing, thinking nothing, trying nothing, and planning nothing has just wasted twenty-four hours. A lot of them balk like irritated camels when I ask them to do the crucially important work of learning to be still. You may be chafing a bit yourself, planning to skip this step and move right on to something "more productive." I put that last phrase in quotation marks because, actually, doing nothing is the most productive activity you will ever undertake. The rest of the Joy Diet can't have its full effect until you have made it a habit.

To do this, you'll have to violate some deeply ingrained cultural rules. We share a powerful collective resistance to nothingness, and feel more virtuous the more somethings we do. You can trace the sociological development of this attitude in Max Weber's classic tome *The Protestant Ethic and the "Spirit" of Capitalism,* which I strongly encourage you not to read, especially if you are a lover of mellifluous prose. Weber observed that the central value of hard, unstinting work—the "Don't just stand there, do something!" approach to life—catalyzed many of our society's phenomenal accomplishments: decoding underlying laws of nature, curing diseases, walking on the moon, inventing the Thighmaster, and so on. No question about it, our cultural obsession with doing something has yielded spectacular results.

The problem is that perpetually doing, without ever tuning in to the center of our being, is the equivalent of fueling a mighty ship by tossing all its navigational equipment into the furnace. Fully occupied by the process of achieving innumerable goals, we lose the ability to determine which goals really matter, and why. Only by connecting with our innate sense of truth can we ensure that the astonishing wealth and power human beings have created will be used for intelligent, benevolent ends. That is why throughout history, everywhere on Earth—even in Max Weber's modern Western Europe—an enormous variety of human cultures have venerated the teachings of a few wise souls who happened to be extremely good at doing nothing.

Nothing Doing: Accounts from the Experts

Mystics, saints, and philosophers consistently tell us that the experience of doing nothing, I mean *really* doing nothing, is impossible to articulate. This is partly because it takes consciousness beyond the reach of verbal thought. Scanning imagery shows that, for example, during meditation, the areas of the brain usually involved in verbal thinking become quiet, and a completely different area "lights up." As this occurs, the meditating person may have a sense of the ego both dissolving and connecting with the entire universe. Chip Brown, a journalist who spent years researching alternative healing, complained that whenever he set out to describe this sensation, he ended up "bludgeoning the ineffable." Perhaps this is why the Buddha's first words upon achieving enlightenment are said to have been, "This cannot be taught." Nevertheless, words can be the vehicles that take us close to the experience of nothing-doing, and some of the human race's most treasured writings include verbal approximations of what it means to add nothing to your life.

For example, ancient Chinese philosophers encouraged seekers to attain a condition known as *mu,* which literally means "uncarved block"—in other words, a something that bears, holds, or represents nothing. Japanese Zen masters use the phrase "the empty mirror," the image in two reflective surfaces set perfectly parallel to one another. This, they say, is your original face, the face you had before your father and mother were born. By returning to it, you can sink the foundations of your character and your actions deep into the radiant stillness that will allow you to handle life's vagaries with wisdom beyond the scope of ego or intellect. Lao Tzu, the father of Taoism, put it this way:

> *We join spokes together in a wheel,*
> *but it is the center hole*
> *that makes the wagon move.*
>
> *We shape clay into a pot,*
> *but it is the emptiness inside*
> *that holds whatever we want.*
>
> *We hammer wood for a house,*
> *but it is the inner space*
> *that makes it livable.*
>
> *We work with being,*
> *but non-being is what we use.*

In case these Asian metaphors aren't ringing your archetypal chimes, you can find the same concept expressed throughout the Muslim and Judeo-Christian traditions. One of my favorites is contained in the Old Testament story of Elijah. This particular prophet was hiding in a cave, muddling over problems that were probably at least as bad as yours (a multiple-murder rap and a gang of would-be executioners), when he heard God calling to him. This is how the Book of Kings describes it:

> *And behold, the Lord passed by, and a great and strong wind tore into the mountains and broke the rocks into pieces before the Lord, but the Lord was not in the wind; and after the wind an earthquake, but the Lord was not in*

*the earthquake; and after the earthquake a fire, but the
Lord was not in the fire; and after the fire a still small voice.*

Even if you've never heard a Bible story, you may recognize
Elijah's experience. In fact, I'd be surprised to learn that you
haven't lived it, in one way or another. Almost all of us have
been assaulted by hurricane winds, rapacious fires, and shatter-
ing earthquakes of some sort; we live on that kind of planet.
Do you remember the last time your preconceptions were
blown to smithereens, your heart burnt to a cinder, your confidence shattered? Look back on it now (or if you're in the middle
of it, look around), and see if in the midst of that devasta-
tion—right in the center of it—you half-sense something still
and small. Listen for it. Beneath, around, even within the
cacophonous chaos of your life disintegrating, something infinitely powerful and surpassingly sweet is whispering to you. It
is when all our somethings are collapsing that we may finally
turn to nothing, and find there everything we need.

Almost everyone seems to use this kind of paradoxical language to describe the effect of doing nothing. Saint John of
the Cross, one of the more eloquent nothing-doers of the
Christian tradition, spoke of traveling to a destination "where,
waiting for me, was the One I knew so well, in that place
where no one ever is." He called the One who met him there
"the beloved," an ambiguous label that certainly meant God,
but could just as accurately mean the true self that was divinely
loved, since in that empty place, the poet wrote, "the lover and
the beloved change bodies."

Whatever metaphor you use to conceptualize the experience of doing nothing, I hope that these brief descriptions
have convinced you it is far more interesting than you may
have been led to believe. If you are currently in any kind of

pain, you may find something oddly compelling about the words of the great nothing-doers. Though they make no logical sense, they have an irrational resonance that sticks to the suffering soul even after the mind has forgotten them, the way nectar remains on your fingertips after you've held a flower.

When Nothing Makes Sense

I myself became interested in nothingness at a particularly stressful time of life. I had grown up firmly opposed to doing nothing, steeped in the American work ethic, positive I could find fulfillment through effort, optimism, stringent calisthenics, and a high-fiber diet. This attitude brought me many good things, but in the end, it proved ineffective at warding off the slings and arrows of outrageous fortune. By my midtwenties, I was utterly exhausted, sick as a mad cow in both body and soul. Chronic pain in my muscles and joints had rendered me almost bedridden. I was working twenty slow, crippled hours a day, trying to revive an academic career that had been mauled nearly to death by the multiple preoccupations of early parenthood. One of my three preschool children had Down syndrome, which meant he would never do many of the somethings I'd always thought were essential for happiness. My life was full to bursting, and yet the more I crammed into my schedule, the more desperately I felt that there was something missing.

I finally became so exhausted that certain words and images began to pierce the armor of my get-things-done belief system. It happened almost against my will; a series of oddly persistent coincidences seemed bent on teaching me how to do nothing. I'd be sorting through textbooks I had used as an undergraduate Chinese major when an odd line of Taoist poetry, something I'd never noticed before, would practically leap off a page and grab me by the hair. On my frequent emergency-room visits, I always seemed to get stuck with the maddeningly flaky doctor who prescribed "mindfulness" instead of the good old-fashioned morphine I'd requested. I felt unexpectedly drawn to people who, once I got to know them, always turned out to have a habit of seeking stillness on a regular basis. It couldn't help but sink in. I gradually learned how to do nothing, though I had no talent or practice. If I can handle the job, trust me, you can too.

How to Do Nothing

A key word in adding nothing to your daily routine is "vacation." Most of us use this word in the phrase "going on vacation," by which we mean traveling to some destination far from home and pursuing recreational activities that may range from gambling to water skiing. This kind of vacation is lovely, as far as it goes, but it can't happen every day, and it won't change the sense that something is missing from your life. In the end, what we've come to call "vacationing" is simply adding a different collection of somethings to our schedules for a brief period. This doesn't meet my favorite definition of "vacation," which is the act of vacating; of leaving, losing touch with, letting go of, a habitual environment. To really do nothing, you must vacate your own life. On the Joy Diet, you do this at least once a day.

Doing Nothing Step 1: Put Up the NO VACANCY Sign

The voice of your true self is so small and still that virtually any distraction can drown it out, especially if you're just beginning to hear it. You simply cannot develop the skill of listening without carving out and vigorously defending chunks of time during which to do nothing. Right now, schedule at least fifteen minutes every day (twenty, if you can get it) for nothing-doing. Then, each day at the appointed time, go to any comfortable, quiet spot. It may be your bedroom, your car, your favorite walking path, the reading room at your local library—pretty much anywhere, as long as you can protect yourself from interruption. For this short time, you must be absolutely unavailable and inaccessible to *everyone*. (I have a nine-dollar watch with an alarm function that I can set to beep at me after my nothing-doing time is up; you can use any kind of timer you prefer.) Let it be known that you are fully occupied, that you have no room for anyone until you have finished doing nothing. Do whatever it takes to light up the NO VACANCY sign on your life.

Many people are shocked when I suggest this. Our culture is becoming more and more obsessed with the ideal, the by-God *duty,* of staying connected no matter what. Cell-phone commercials show supposedly "vacationing" businessmen closing deals from pristine wilderness lakes. Television news feeds us as many as five information streams at a time (the anchorperson, stock ticker, factoid bubbles, weather report, and running captions). The average white-collar worker receives about 230 messages a day via a cornucopia of communication technologies. Every new way to connect brings a fresh set of demands on our limited attention—and how do we try to cope with the overwhelm? Why, of course, by inventing still more ways to stay connected! Our societal belief is that we can solve the problem of overcommitment by using more gadgets to do more things more quickly and efficiently. This is like trying to dig your way out of a pit. Many of us are reaching the point of attention burnout.

This is certainly familiar territory for yours truly. Those rare periods when I answer all my e-mail always end with me hunched at my computer, muttering and rocking like Rain Man when he couldn't get cheese puffs. The relief I feel when I send off the last message crumbles the next time I log on to my computer and read, "Welcome! You have one hundred and six unread messages!" The nine phone calls and twelve letters that came in while I was online don't help matters. Eventually, my ability to process all the demands on my attention disintegrates, and I spend entire days doing what cartoonist Scott Adams calls "multi-shirking," just sitting around feeling guilty about all the connections I'm not sustaining.

If this ever happens to you, the fact is that you're probably already making yourself unavailable to everyone in your life for at least half an hour a day, possibly much longer. Your deep self knows that you need much more nothing, and whenever you won't consciously put up the NO VACANCY sign, it tries to help by sabotaging your ability to concentrate, to communicate, to connect. I suggest that instead of spending your idle time stewing in guilt, you do nothing, with pride and gusto. For that precious quarter of an hour, trust that it is all right to close your literal and figurative doors to everyone but yourself. If people ask where you're going, tell them the truth: that you have an extremely important meeting scheduled. You needn't reveal that the meeting is in "the place where no one ever is," with the One who waits for you there. They might not understand that missing this particular meeting would have a more deleterious effect on your life than any other form of disconnection.

Doing Nothing Step 2: Let Your Body Vacate

Once you've established the condition of NO VACANCY, you'll become paradoxically free to vacate—that is, to let go of everything in your life except the awareness of your own soul. This process begins with the body. Technically, of course, you can't force your body to do nothing; until you pass away, your heart will keep beating, your ears hearing, your nose picking up smells. The way your body can help you vacate is by engaging in physical actions that create inner stillness, rather than distraction.

There are several ways you might do this. These days, I often use traditional meditation, which begins with simply sitting down and relaxing into physical stillness. However, this didn't always work for me, and it may not be the best approach for you. If you have suffered greatly and not yet resolved your pain, you may find it literally unbearable to become physically still; the moment you really quiet your body, you'll feel the monsters of unprocessed grief, rage, or fear yammering at the dungeon doors of your subconscious mind. This can trigger an intense fight/flight reaction, flooding your body with adrenaline that will render you angry, anxious, or restless, rather than peaceful.

Physical movement allows your body to respond to this hormonal surge, so if sitting still feels unbearable, I recommend any mindless, repetitive motion to keep your body busy while you do nothing. Go for a level of activity that allows you to move rhythmically without having to struggle, pant, or concentrate on keeping yourself moving. Walking, jogging, swimming, Rollerblading, and driving have all worked for me at various times. So have martial-arts kicking or punching drills (I especially recommend this for people who may have just a smidgen of repressed rage, though of course I never did). If your body is tired, seek out some fluidly moving part of nature: a fireplace, a river, a field of wind-blown wheat, a thundering surf. Watching and listening to the patterned disorder of the universe is one of the deep soul's favorite pastimes. The important thing is that whatever physical action you choose requires no deliberate thought; you can do it without any conscious attention at all.

Doing Nothing Step 3: Vacate Your Mind

You've probably heard the phrase "I think, therefore I am." This statement came from René Descartes, a philosopher who helped articulate our good friend, Western European rationalism. It is rumored that Descartes died an unusual death: When the hostess at a tea party offered him sugar, he said, "I think not," and immediately disappeared. All right, the joke is lame, but it does express one of our society's core beliefs: that to think is to exist, that our analytical minds constitute our fundamental identity. This is an illusion that can cause immeasurable suffering. On the Joy Diet, you have to see through it, if only for a few minutes a day.

Once you have set aside time and quieted your body (either by stillness or motion), turn your attention to whatever is happening in your mind. There's probably a lot going on in there. The typical human mind is like a supercomputer possessed by the soul of a demented squirrel. It's constantly calculating, anticipating, remembering, fantasizing, worrying, hoarding, bouncing frenetically from thought to thought to thought. My own mind is so manic that all my life, people have given me advice about how to calm it down. "Breathe deeply," they tell me. "Listen to soothing music. Stop thinking." Oh, sure. I might as well try to stop growing hair. I can sit around hyperventilating to the strains of Enya until the cows, goats, and migratory birds come home, and my mind still churns out thoughts like a malfunctioning Twinkie extruder.

If you're one of those enlightened people who can simply stop thinking for fifteen minutes a day, go for it. If you have a squirrel brain like mine, however, an easier option—in fact, your only option—is to simply watch your mind do its thing, without passing any judgments on your thoughts, or trying to control the process. The act of nonjudgmental observation is extremely powerful, allowing you to divide your awareness from your thoughts. A writer named Sri Nisargadatta Maharaj puts it this way:

> *Know yourself to be the changeless witness of the changeful mind. Mind is interested in what happens, while the awareness is interested in the mind itself. The child is after the toy, but the mother watches the child not the toy.*

There are many techniques to help you detach from the restless, wandering child that is your mind, and become the kind, nonjudgmental mother who regards that child with tolerant affection. You may be familiar with (or partial to) some traditional meditation techniques, most of which include focusing on your breath or a mantra, clearing your mind, and gently shooing away distracting thoughts. The methods I use most often are slightly different from these, in that there is a bit more verbal activity happening in the brain when you do them. They all share two very simple elements: watching and naming. Here are a few you might try.

THE TICKER TAPE

Once your body is on vacation and you've tuned in to your mind, imagine that your thoughts are being written down on a ticker tape that streams across your field of vision from left to right (or right to left, if your thoughts happen to be in Hebrew). Don't edit or control what your mind says, just read it. "My head hurts," the ticker tape may say. "I'm sure I have a brain tumor." "I'm going to die." "And nobody will care." "I should update my will." As each thought goes by, silently describe it with a word or short phrase: "Pain." "Thinking." "Fear." "Worry." Etc., etc., etc.

THE ONE CHAIR

If ticker tape doesn't work for you, you might try the traditional practice called "taking the one chair." Imagine yourself sitting on the only seat in an empty room. Watch your thoughts go by in front of you, as images, words, or feelings. Remember that since you've taken the only chair, there's no room for any of these mind products to stay. Watch and name them as they pass by, then let them leave the "room."

THE WATERFALL

If your mind is particularly rambunctious, say, during a time when life is turbulent and scary, picture yourself entering a small cave behind a thundering waterfall. Stay there in the cool spray and watch the contents of your mind thunder past you like falling water. Whenever a thought or feeling becomes clear, name it. If things are moving too fast to label, just watch and notice that no matter how violent the downpour, you are able to sit apart from it.

THE PARADE

Attending a parade is a fine thing to do on vacation, something I indulge in frequently without even opening my eyes. On any given day, the parade in my brain includes a wide variety of interesting attractions: mundane logistical thoughts that plod past me like the marchers in a high school band; silly thoughts that tumble through my head like clowns; noble thoughts striding along magnificently, like the Budweiser Clydesdales; and humble thoughts that follow the Clydesdales to shovel up their inevitable load of crap. I don't judge or control the elements of my thought procession; just as with the other techniques, I simply call them by name and watch them move on by.

If you practice any or all of these techniques every day, you'll slowly become aware of an underlying calm that is always present within you, even when your thoughts and emotions are in an uproar. In fact, you'll find that moods and worries begin to move through you, instead of sticking around to dominate your life. Even on the days when doing nothing feels flat and stupid, you'll notice it makes the rest of your life less frightening and more manageable. You'll gradually learn by actual experience that your thoughts are not you, that thinking is not the process by which you recognize the keys to your existence, things like beauty, truth, and love. That role belongs to the One Who Knows, the wise silence that is the ground of your real self and the source of your real joy.

Doing Nothing Step 4: Learn to Return

When I was just beginning to practice doing nothing, I had a chance to spend several days in a place off the coast of Thailand called Amanpuri, which is Sanskrit for "The Place of Peace." I occupied a small hut in an abandoned coconut plantation, where monkeys and parrots called above me and the ocean breathed below. My room had no television, no telephone, no e-mail access, and no visitors. On my first day there, after about six hours of having nothing to do, I thought I'd go out of my mind. I'm glad to report that's exactly what happened. By the third day, my mind had separated from my sense of self so gently and completely that I began to forget exactly why I usually wear clothes.

Nowadays, when I sit down to do nothing, it helps to begin by remembering the Amanpuri. I recall the still, humid air of the jungle, the rush of the surf, the feeling of being a thousand miles from anywhere. This triggers a reaction psychologists call "state-dependent memory." What this means is that when we reenter an old environment, we are likely to remember, very vividly, the thoughts and feelings we experienced the last time we were there. By picturing my place of peace, I can quickly recapture at least the echo of the complete relaxation I experienced in my little seaside home.

I highly recommend that you locate or create your own Amanpuri, a mental "place of peace" where you go to meet the Beloved. If you have any memories of peace and stillness, call them up as you begin your daily dose of nothing-doing. Remember, really remember, what it felt like that moment you stood alone on a mountaintop, or played baseball in ankle-deep grass, or lost yourself in music. If your life has been so unremittingly awful that you can't recall any peaceful scenes, create an imaginary place that feels safe. I know a former battered wife whose place of peace is an imaginary space capsule a million miles from the earth (which she considers a very dangerous location).

Whatever your Amanpuri is like, visit it only when you are doing nothing. Once you come to associate it with stepping away from your mind, it will make the process quicker and more enjoyable. It will also make you aware that your life can be blessed by a constant undercurrent of love, even in the midst of suffering. When you first add nothing to your schedule, you may fear that you're courting the kind of torpor that turns lazy people into abject failures. But the more nothing you do, the more you will see that there has always been, and always will be, a part of you that accomplishes more with stillness than you could with frenzied action. As the poet Antonio Machado puts it,

> *My soul is not asleep! My soul is not asleep!*
> *It neither sleeps nor dreams, but watches, its clear eyes open,*
> *far off things, and listens, and listens*
> *at the shores of the great silence.*
> *It listens at the shores of the great silence.*

What our souls hear, when we finally surrender to the great silence, is the next element of the Joy Diet.

MENU ITEM #1: NOTHING
MINIMUM DAILY REQUIREMENTS

At least once a day:

1. Put up the NO VACANCY sign. Set aside fifteen minutes every day when you will not be bothered by *anybody,* for *anything.*

2. Let your body vacate.
>Option one: Sit quietly and allow your body to relax.
>Option two: Engage in any repetitive, mindless physical activity.
>Option three: Find a place to watch some natural motion, such as fire or running water.

3. Vacate your mind. Detach from your thoughts by watching them. Visualize them as written words on ticker tape, a stream of traffic in a room, a waterfall, a parade, or any other procession of words and objects.

4. Learn to return. Create a strong, vivid memory of a place where you felt utterly at ease. Return there mentally whenever you do nothing.

TRUTH

•

CREATE AND ABSORB AT LEAST ONE MOMENT
OF TRUTH EACH DAY.

"WHEREVER YOU GO," SAYS THE POPULAR ADAGE, "THERE you are." To you this may sound like an unassailably accurate statement. Not to me. Most of the people I coach—most of the people I *know*—don't spend much of their time where they are. I certainly don't. Of course, it's true that since going on the Joy Diet, I experience daily moments, even hours, of being where I am; fully and completely present in the space and time I occupy right here and now. But I spend at least as much time visiting faraway locations like What If and Should Be and I Wonder When and If Only. . . . In other words, my mind is often focused on circumstances that only exist in my fears, hopes, and fantasies, to the point where I disengage from much of what I am actually experiencing.

There's nothing wrong with this; dissociation is an astonishingly useful psychological mechanism, one I've found to be lifesaving when I'm undergoing something unbearable, such as severe illness or a PTA meeting. However, it's possible to get stuck in a mental zone that offers virtually no access to genuine experience. When this happens, we become strangely unable to really see, smell, touch, taste, and hear life as it happens to us. Our senses work, but our hearts don't feel connected to them. Virginia Woolf described this as "living behind a pane of glass" and found it so intolerable that one day she filled her pockets with rocks and took a terminal stroll into the Thames. Having spent several years behind a psychological windowpane myself, I don't blame her. But I do wish Virginia had been able to break through to a life of connection and joy by committing a different kind of suicide: the ego death that comes when we allow ourselves to live in complete, compassionate accord with what we know and feel to be the truth.

Growing up in Utah, a state chock-full o' religious enthusiasts, I heard the phrase "the truth will set you free" quite often. It was usually followed by phrases that contained capitalized words, such as "Ours is the One True Church," or "We know the Plan of Salvation." As an obsequiously high-achieving child, I earnestly believed all these things, then waited for the thrill of spiritual liberation. Sometimes I thought I felt a vague inner stirring, but nothing intense enough to make me sure it wasn't just gas. It wasn't until years later that I realized I'd been groping for the wrong truths, that in my humble case, the liberation of the soul comes not from theological proclamations, but from the simple truths of basic experience: This is what I love. This is what I need. This is what makes me angry. This is what's happening, right now.

Menu Item #2 of the Joy Diet consists of telling yourself this kind of truth at least once a day. I'll explain how in this chapter. First, you'll conduct a tiny, underfunded research campaign by asking and answering a few specific questions. These questions are very simple, and I guarantee you'll always have the information you need to answer them correctly (though you may not realize it). Next you'll create an environment of compassion where the truths you tell will lead to deeper and deeper levels of awareness. The whole thing can be accomplished in about two or three minutes, but that brief interlude can improve your life more than you'd believe.

Why We Hide from the Truth

The practice of telling ourselves the truth is so simple and so freeing that you'd think we'd all do it constantly. The fact is, however, that most people tell themselves the truth only in selected areas, and many of us lie to ourselves and others about practically everything we experience. Why? Because living behind a pane of glass, numbing and empty though it is, also feels safe.

The Inner Effect of Truth

My client Delilah had decided to break up with her abusive boyfriend of ten years. She alternated between rock-solid determination and fainthearted second-guessing.

"Maybe I'm making a huge mistake," she said one day. "What if I leave, and then I'm not happy without him?"

"Could happen," I said. "But tell me, have you ever been happy *with* him?"

"Oh, yes," said Delilah very earnestly. "It hasn't been all that bad. There used to be lots of times when I didn't realize how miserable I was."

This sorry little reward—unawareness of our pain—is the payoff we get for failing to tell ourselves the disturbing truths we already know. It seems like a pathetic excuse for happiness, until you're the one looking through the soothing haze of self-deception only to catch glimpses of a terrifying truth that demands enormous change.

There's an old fairy tale about a giant who, in an attempt to become immortal, puts his heart in a container like one of those nested Russian dolls: dozens of boxes inside of boxes inside of boxes. Then he buries the whole assembly in a deep hole far from his home. After that, no matter what his enemies do, they can't kill the giant, because nothing ever comes within a country mile of his heart. The catch is that he achieves his invulnerability at the cost of his capacity to love, to feel, to enjoy. The giant is physically alive, but emotionally dead. When the hero finally digs up the boxes, opens all of them, and destroys the giant's heart, it feels like a mercy killing.

This tale is a metaphor for the way we humans hide our hearts from pain. Sigmund Freud, who in my opinion was wrong about many things, was right about this: Human beings are able to bury unpleasant, frightening, or forbidden truths in our subconscious minds so effectively that our conscious selves literally don't know what we know or feel what we feel. This is what psychologists call denial, and although it masquerades as ignorance, it's actually the opposite. Ironically, the things we refuse to know are by definition things we know already—that's how we know we don't want to know them, y'know?

Because we are so blind to the things we don't want to see, other people are often on to us long before we ourselves even suspect the truth about what we know and feel. I've learned to expect that clients who exude rage will tell me they've never felt angry in their lives. The most manically effervescent people are often filled with bottomless despair. I've had half a dozen clients who have described their secret extramarital affairs, then hotly criticized their spouses for lacking their high level of emotional openness and honesty. This astonishing ability to keep from seeing the obvious is necessary for us to preserve our image of ourselves. Denial only becomes stronger when other people are involved.

The Outer Effect of Truth

Without exception, denial is a tool we haul out when the truth would rock the various social boats in which we live our lives. The things we hide from ourselves are realities that, if we actually experienced them, would threaten our status quo, bring us into conflict with the systems we depend on, and fling us into the unknown. The truth threatens everything about us that is not authentic: every habit, every relationship, every financial arrangement, every belief.

I know whereof I speak. On New Year's Day, 1992, I made just one resolution: I wouldn't lie, not once, for the entire year. A few months later, when I desperately sought out a therapist to help me cope with the fact that my life had exploded, she told me my problem was that I keep my New Year's resolutions. She was joking, but she was right. My little truth-telling commitment had set me on a course that would lead me away from almost everything I thought defined me: my job, my profession, my religion, my home, and pretty much every relationship I'd ever formed before the age of about twenty.

Here's one example of the many ways I got to test my resolution resolve. I was living in Utah at the time, raising my kids and teaching while I wrote my dissertation. Since my field of study was the sociology of gender, I was studying gender relations in the predominant local religion, which I will not name here (press the buzzer when you have the right answer). I occasionally got calls from reporters asking for comments about this topic. Common sense said to stay out of these troubled political waters, but I believed Aleksandr Solzhenitsyn's statement that "there are times when silence is a lie." So I was usually willing to tell inquiring journalists things I knew from research, such as the percentage of local women who were employed or the number of divorces in the Utah community. Elsewhere, these would be considered mundane statistics; in this particular fertile crescent, they were hand grenades. I got a lot of none-too-subtle feedback, such as anonymous hate mail and threatening phone calls. One day a local religious leader came to my house and told me outright that I had to stop making "inappropriate" statements.

"Here's my position," I told him carefully (I spoke more slowly than usual that year, trying to make sure before it came out of my mouth that everything I said was really true). "I respect the people who run this church. So far as I know, they're very good men. But if one of them told me to do something that I believed in my heart to be wrong, I wouldn't do it."

He sighed uncomfortably. "Well, I understand," he said. "But if you ever say that publicly, we'll have to take action against you. And by the way, terrible things happen to children in this town whose parents aren't in good standing with The Church. We can't control what happens to yours."

In retrospect, this seems bizarre and creepy, like being targeted for assassination by the Brady Bunch (actually, come to think of it, that's exactly how it felt at the time). But you see my point, right? My truth-telling was not copacetic with the prevailing social system. This caused me some curious confrontations, unpleasant disagreements, and nervous nights. Above all, it brought me loss after loss after loss, as different individuals and groups severed their relationships with me.

Common sense said to put a sock in all this truth stuff, to just keep my nice, orderly life the way it had been before. But I didn't—couldn't—because for all I was losing, I was finding something that mattered more. "What does it profit a man," Jesus is supposed to have said, "if he should gain the whole world, and lose his own soul?" In 1992 and the years that followed, I realized that the simple, small truths of my real thoughts and experiences were the keys that unlocked the dungeon doors for my true self. Trying to stop telling them would have been like trying to give up oxygen.

This was an almost inexpressibly painful period of my life, but as it drew on, I began to feel intensely, vividly alive. Prior to that time, I'd had no idea so much joy was even possible. I've watched with pain and pride as dozens of my clients have taken the same kind of plunge, determining to tell themselves the truth, no matter what, then opening up secret after secret, breaking through lie by lie, until they find their hearts. I only recommend that they go for one Moment of Truth a day, but the effect is the same whether you go for broke, as I did, or proceed more gradually, as I suggest. As far as I can tell, this process is always hard, always painful, always so, so worth it.

How to Create Your Daily Moment of Truth

If you did nothing but pursue the truth about yourself for the rest of your life, you would never run out of fresh discoveries. Every day brings you new experiences, changing you, bringing new aspects of your true self into expression. There are so many layers of thought and perception in your mind, so many interactive connections that have been developing from infancy on, that the largest part of you will always be an undiscovered country. As you tell fewer fibs and keep fewer secrets in your inner world, you'll find that the energy you once spent on denial turns outward in a kind of creative bloom. Fascinating ideas, compassionate actions, unheard-of adventures will bubble up from the inexhaustible well of your unique personality during your Moments of Truth. The procedure for creating all this excitement is very simple.

Truth Step 1: Start with Your Daily Dose of Nothing

If you can't get yourself to do Menu Item #1 (nothing), you're not ready for Menu Item #2. The thing that most consistently makes us resist doing nothing is our hidden awareness of some truth our conscious minds find too threatening to tolerate. It's actually quite difficult to keep such knowledge out of consciousness, because the truths that can set us free are not inert. They want to be told, to be known. They are constantly pushing outward toward consciousness, popping into our dreams, sidling into our suspicions, and popping out in Freudian slips. We have to push back, hard, to continue not knowing them. We use all kinds of techniques: muscle tension, constant work, addiction, obsession, compulsive behaviors of all kinds.

All of these repressive techniques are the work of the body and/or the conscious mind. When we still both, there is nothing to fight the progress of liberating truths into our consciousness. This is why stillness often makes us feel edgy, or bored, or unbearably confined—fifteen minutes of calm relaxation, in and of itself, wouldn't create such intense resistance. If you find yourself becoming intensely annoyed by the thought of doing nothing for fifteen minutes, if the very thought alarms, nauseates, or otherwise repels you, then you are hiding something from yourself. As a wise man once said, you can't handle the truth. Well, that's all right. Until and unless you reach the point where a few minutes of stillness becomes tolerable, you can substitute a preliminary primer question for Menu Item #2. Every day, at least once, ask and answer this question:

> ### PRIMER QUESTION FOR MENU ITEM #2
>
> Why am I avoiding stillness?

You don't have to list a catalog of childhood traumas or mental blocks; we're not looking for anything that complicated. A simple "Because I don't like it" will do nicely, *as long as it is the honest-to-goodness truth.* Continue to ask and answer this same question every day, until you are able to tolerate a full quarter hour of doing nothing. If you're honest, you'll find that you give slightly different responses on different days: "Because stillness makes me anxious." "Because it pisses me off." "Because it's a waste of time." "Because I'm afraid." Whatever the answer is, simply acknowledge it, and your Moment of Truth will be complete.

The thing about denial is that any form of truth directed at it dissolves it, the way a solvent dissolves grease. If you're afraid to know what you know and feel what you feel, simply acknowledging your fear begins to erode your denial. (Handy hint: You can also use the solvent of acknowledgment on the unexpressed truths that tend to accrete around relationship problems. If you're nervous about being open with someone— say, for example, you're in love or angry with them, and don't feel confident expressing these emotions—you can begin to melt the impasse by saying, "There's something I'd like to talk to you about, but it makes me really nervous." Articulating the fear is always the best first step to getting past it.)

Truth Step 2: Once You've Learned to Do Nothing, Ask and Answer These Questions Daily

Once you get to the point where you can handle stillness, you're ready for the question-and-answer session that will create your Moment of Truth. After fifteen minutes of nothing, ask and answer this:

FIRST DAILY QUESTION FOR MENU ITEM #2

What am I feeling?

Let the answer come by itself, in a stream of consciousness. Often, your first answers will be descriptions of physical sensations: "My nose itches." "I'm hot." "I'm tired." Sometimes that's where the answers will end. More often, though, your responses will come in layers, different feelings rising through your consciousness like bubbles rising through water. Let them all come. Let your true self tell its story, while your mind provides the narration. *Don't explain the feelings. Just describe them.*

When I ask new clients what they're feeling, they almost always launch into a discourse about whatever they're thinking. Watch out for this tendency when you're doing Menu Item #2. "I feel that the Republicans are ruining this country" is not an expression of a sensation; it's just a thought dressed in the language of feeling. The real truth might be "I feel scared and angry," or "My father is a Republican, and I hate him."

It is crucial that you not censor or judge the realities of your emotional experience. There is no such thing as an evil or stupid feeling, though we sometimes do evil and stupid things in response to our feelings. We're in far more danger of doing this when we deny or minimize our darker impulses than when we accept them honestly and fully. A therapist I know, a compassionate soul who radiates acceptance and wouldn't hurt a gnat, freely admits to having homicidal impulses during meditation. She once referred me to this poem by the Sufi poet Rumi.

> *This being human is a guest house.*
> *Every morning a new arrival.*
>
> *A joy, a depression, a meanness,*
> *some momentary awareness comes*
> *as an unexpected visitor.*
>
> *Welcome and entertain them all!*
> *Even if they're a crowd of sorrows,*
> *who violently sweep your house*
> *empty of its furniture,*
> *still, treat each guest honorably.*
> *He may be clearing you out*
> *for some new delight.*
>
> *The dark thought, the shame, the malice,*
> *meet them at the door laughing,*
> *and invite them in.*

If you make a habit of this, you'll find that your "bad" feelings are exactly the ones that you most need to explore. The feeling you think is bad beyond belief may be the only teacher in the universe from whom you can learn genuine goodness. If you continue to ask patiently, without trying to control your feelings, they will lead you to the naturally loving being that is your true self. Rage will melt away to reveal fear, which will gradually show itself as a need to freely love and be loved. Jealousy will soften into sadness, then compassion. Just watch. Then move on to the next question.

SECOND DAILY QUESTION FOR MENU ITEM #2

What hurts?

It may be that there is absolutely nothing wrong with you today, in which case the honest answer is "Nothing." It may be that the answer is "My leg," or "My right ear," in which case you should stretch out a bit, or see a doctor, or do whatever else it takes to make your leg or your right ear feel better. Unless you're way more enlightened than I am, however, your suffering won't always end with physical pain. Usually, there will be something in your emotions, your figurative belly, that is upsetting, disgruntling, or maybe just irksome. Good! These inner discomforts are wonderful opportunities to find out deeper truths about the habits of mind that are causing you to suffer.

If you do discover that you are suffering emotional pain of any kind—worry, grief, fury, shame, hate, dejection, take your pick—don't fight it. Sit there and let the feeling grow as big as it wants to be. Let it fill your whole universe, if that's what it decides to do. Let it tell you all the terrifying or enraging or devastating details of whatever situation engendered it. Then ask yourself this:

THIRD DAILY QUESTION FOR MENU ITEM #2

What is the painful story I'm telling?

At first, your pain may seem to come from nowhere, but if you poke around with the question "What hurts?," you'll eventually start associating your pain with memories or concerns for the future. The ache in your heart will stir up recollections of an old boyfriend. Your anger will really get rolling as the image of your office manager minces into your mind. If you pay attention, you'll find that there are beliefs connected to these images, axioms so familiar and well-rehearsed that they feel like good, solid, carved-in-stone facts.

> *"He never really loved me. No one ever has. I'm too fat, that's the problem. I'm too fat too fat too fat too fat too fat. . . ."*

> *"She's a nasty, horrible person, and she's going to get me fired, just like she got Bob fired. There's nothing I can do about it. I have to suck up to that bitch. . . ."*

> *"I'll never be able to finish all the work I have to do this week. It will be horrible. I'll have to work so hard, and I won't get any sleep, and I'll get in trouble. . . ."*

And so on.

Therapists from a branch of psychology called ACT (short for Acceptance and Commitment Theory) coined the terms "clean pain" and "dirty pain" to refer to suffering that comes from real events, as opposed to suffering that comes from the stories we tell ourselves about those events. Clean pain comes when we suffer a loss or injury, such as the death of a loved one or the physical discomfort of sickness. Dirty pain is caused by what we think about these events—or other events that may involve no real injury at all. If you're a typical human, you'll find that dirty pain outweighs clean pain in your life by a huge margin. In other words, most of your pain comes not from reality, but from your stories about reality. Once you've located one of them, ask yourself:

FOURTH DAILY QUESTION FOR MENU ITEM #2

Can I be sure my painful story is true?

Dostoevsky wrote that the best way to keep a prisoner from escaping is to make sure he never knows he's in prison. Many of us live this way, not even knowing how desperately we are trapped by the stories we tell to make sense of our experience. Once these stories are in place, we choose, modify, and twist new experiences to fit our expectations. What we think of as the "truth" is actually an elaborate and deliberate fiction composed by our own minds. Realizing that your story is really arbitrary, that there are infinite other stories that may be every bit as accurate, opens the prison door of your belief system, allowing you to walk out if you so choose.

Your initial response to the question "Is my painful story true?" will probably be a knee-jerk "Yes! Of course!" So speaks the voice of illusion. Sit with the question for a while, and you'll begin to see that your stories are impossible to verify absolutely, because they're based on subjective perceptions. René Descartes, whom we met in the last chapter, once sat up all night fussing about the fact that there was no way he could tell for sure that he wasn't just dreaming everything he thought of as reality. The Chinese philosopher Chuang Tzu put it more poetically. "Last night," he said, "I dreamt I was a butterfly, and today I don't know whether I was a man dreaming he was a butterfly, or whether I am now a butterfly dreaming he is a man." The point is that there's virtually nothing of which anyone can be utterly positive. In fact, I can think of only two reliable certainties any of us can claim: the reality of our existence, and the fact that no matter what we believe, we could be wrong. Unless I'm wrong.

Anyway, acknowledging that we don't—can't—know the Absolute Truth may not be a particularly comfortable thought, but it is incredibly liberating. It opens closed minds, hearts, and fists faster than any other realization. It allows us to learn from ongoing experience, which is why Plato wrote that we gain our first measure of intelligence when we admit our own ignorance. Once we begin living with the full awareness of our basic fallibility, we can regain what Buddhists call the "don't-know mind," the alert, receptive mental state that makes us capable of genuine perception.

Author and teacher Byron Katie learned this dramatically in her early forties, when she ended decades of rage, depression, and self-hatred by addressing her mind's stories with intense inquiry about the real truth of her experience. In her wonderfully useful book *Loving What Is,* Katie describes how this worked on a night when her daughter, who at the time was abusing drugs and alcohol, failed to come home.

> *The thoughts that would appear in my mind were thoughts like these: '. . . she'll drive, and she'll kill someone, she'll crash into another car or a lamppost and kill herself and her passengers.' As the thoughts appeared, each one was met with wordless, thoughtless inquiry. And inquiry instantly brought me back to reality. Here is what was true: woman sitting in chair waiting for her beloved daughter.*

Katie's method of inquiry, which I highly recommend, requires that you identify painful issues in your own life, examine the stories you tell yourself about the situation, and notice that these stories often have little to do with the "clean pain" of genuine experience. This alone may begin to ease your suffering. You can accentuate the effect by asking:

FIFTH DAILY QUESTION FOR MENU ITEM #2

Is my painful story working?

By "is my story working?" I mean, is your story helping you to feel peaceful, balanced, and able to face life's difficulties by growing and changing? My own belief (which of course, I can't prove) is that our core selves are truth-detection machines that thrive on reality and pine away when fed a diet of misunderstanding. Most people assume that we feel good when we believe pleasant thoughts, and bad when we believe unpleasant ones, but my observations of myself, my loved ones, and my clients don't bear out that assumption. I think deep-seated, long-lasting, intractable emotional pain is always evidence that we believe something false.

For example, my client LeeAnn couldn't begin to get over her divorce as long as she believed her ex-husband's claim that he had never loved her. A year after their breakup, LeeAnn's ex called her to say he'd started therapy, and he wanted her to know that although they did have irreconcilable differences, he had indeed loved her very deeply. Suddenly, LeeAnn's feelings of craziness and mistrust disappeared, and the pain of the divorce itself began to heal almost tangibly. On the other hand, I had a young client named Clint whose father once told him,

"I've always hated you. I don't even believe you're mine." Clint's reaction to these awful statements was a feeling of sadness, but also deep peace and serenity. He had always felt the truth about his father's feelings toward him, and trying to pretend that he had a normal, caring dad had almost driven him nuts. The truth, even the hard truth, is something our core selves can deal with. Believing lies causes us to suffer immeasurably, motivating us to question our beliefs until we can clear up our misperceptions. So the last question you need to complete your Moment of Truth is:

SIXTH DAILY QUESTION FOR MENU ITEM #2

Can I think of another story that might work better?

Byron Katie's method of inquiry involves something she calls a "turnaround." To do it, you just change your story by stating its opposite, or switching the subject and the object, and seeing if the resulting story feels as true or truer than the original.

The first time I tried this, I was frustrated because I'd injured my knee and couldn't continue a rather ambitious exercise program I'd just begun. There was some "clean pain" in my knee, but most of my suffering was "dirty." It came from my frustration with having to stop working out, my belief that my injury would cause me to simultaneously atrophy and blimp up like an emergency life raft. My mental story, which I had written down, was, "I'm furious because I want my knee to heal, so that I can work out like I'm supposed to." When I reversed the story, it became, "I'm furious because my knee wants me to heal, so that I can't work out, like I'm not supposed to."

When I read this back to myself, I laughed out loud. Every part of me resonated to this new story. Suddenly, I noticed several things I'd been hiding behind a wall of denial: the fact that I was tired, that I knew my new exercise program was too rigorous for me, and that I was damaging myself by trying to exceed my physical limits. This realization didn't change the pain in my knee, but all the "dirty" pain around it disappeared. I honestly felt grateful to my injury for helping me find my sense of balance. This probably helped me heal faster physically, though I no longer felt any urgency about that.

Reversing your story may or may not have this effect on you. But if you identify a story that is associated with emotional pain, keep trying different permutations and explanations for it until you feel the open, satisfying sense that you've stumbled upon a story more true than the one you've been using to hurt yourself. This brings us back full circle to our original question, "What am I feeling?" In the end, this is a far more accurate gauge of what is real and true than anything our brains can manufacture. As the Asian proverb puts it, the mind is a wonderful servant, but a terrible master. Put your heart in charge of the question–and–answer session that comprises most of your Moment of Truth.

Truth Step 3: Offer Compassion to Your Inner Lying Scumbag

Whether you've just barely been able to face the primer question, or whether you've zipped through your Moment of Truth to arrive at some pivotal realization, you should finish Menu Item #2 by offering yourself a large serving of compassion. My clients seem to benefit most from classic "loving-kindness" meditations. These are very simple. Breathe deeply, and with each breath, silently repeat compassionate phrases: "May I be happy. May I be well. May I be free from suffering." You certainly deserve these wishes after seeking the truth— something many people wouldn't do if you paid them a fortune and threatened their lives to boot. Continue offering yourself compassion for several breaths, and again throughout the day whenever it occurs to you.

This is particularly crucial if you have discovered that a part of you is in deep denial, or that you can't tolerate even a moment of stillness, or that you are an unscrupulous drug addict who customarily cheats, steals, and willfully offends small animals. The dirtiest, most low-down part of you is the part to which you must offer your compassion, because this person is in fact a wounded and terrified child. He or she has adopted bad habits in a misguided attempt to make the world feel safe. Love and understanding will create a climate where you won't need to take any drastic or immoral action to ensure your safety, and eliminate the need for your "bad" self to go on being bad.

Mind you, this is very, very different from condoning the atrocious things we can do when we let our wounded-child selves rule our behavior. Just because you're scared or sad doesn't give you carte blanche to rage at your family, stuff down four full-size pizzas, lie to your boss, bite the ear off your boxing opponent, or let your demons run wild in other harmful ways. In fact, recognizing the source of your behavior gives you the responsibility—that is, the response-ability—to care for your frightened, damaged aspects in ways that will not harm you or others. Career counselor Richard Bolles recommends that you consider your possible options with just one criterion in mind:

ACTION CRITERION FOR MENU ITEM #2

Of the options open to me, which one brings the most love into the world?

If you think there is no action that you can perform in your current circumstances that will increase the supply of love in the world, you are believing a lie. You will probably feel dark and crazy until you test it against reality. At the very least, you always have the option to offer yourself kindness and understanding. That alone can increase the supply of love in the world. May you be well. May you be happy. May you be free from suffering.

Victor Frankl, a survivor of the Nazi death camps, said, "There are two ways to go to the gas chamber: free or not free." It is the truth that offers us this freedom, the freedom to test what we are taught, to accept what we feel in our hearts, to believe what we know in our bones, and to love ourselves—including the worst aspects of ourselves—until we see through enough of our illusions to discover who we were really meant to be. At that point, we will have dismantled the biggest lie, the most profound denial of all: the denial of our own inestimable power and value. As Marianne Williamson puts it, "Our deepest fear is not that we are inadequate. Our deepest fear is that we are powerful beyond measure. It is our light, not our darkness, that frightens us." Once you've awakened to this light, you will gradually, almost involuntarily, begin to act more like yourself—not out of a desire to attack anyone else's truth, but simply because you cannot un-see what you have seen. Without your having to force it or try or even hope, the truth will set you free.

MENU ITEM #2: TRUTH

MINIMUM DAILY REQUIREMENTS

At least once a day:

1. Start with your daily dose of nothing. If you can't cope with doing nothing, you can fulfill your requirements by asking and answering the question "Why am I avoiding stillness?"

2. Ask and answer these questions.
What am I feeling?
What hurts?
What is the painful story I'm telling?
Can I be sure my painful story is true?
Is my painful story working?
Can I think of another story that might work better?

3. Offer compassion to your inner lying scumbag. As you breathe in and out, offer loving wishes to the parts of yourself that seem to deserve it least.

DESIRE

•

**EACH DAY, IDENTIFY, ARTICULATE, AND EXPLORE
AT LEAST ONE OF YOUR HEART'S DESIRES.**

ONE OF THE MOST AMAZING THINGS ABOUT YOUR BODY IS that the instructions for assembling it, from random protein molecules you can find around the house, are coded into every one of your trillion-plus cells. They are spelled out on the elegant double helix of your DNA, which will preserve your physical identity throughout life, even as it continuously replaces all the actual particles that comprise you and makes sure that you change dramatically from infancy through puberty and all the way to old age. Though environmental factors can alter the structure of your body, your basic physiological identity is permanently and indelibly integrated into your fundamental being.

I happen to believe that the same thing is true of your life—or, to put it more romantically, your destiny. I think we're all born with a set of preferred activities and talents, but more than that, with an inexplicable inner knowledge of the things we are meant to do and be, the changes we are meant to make in the world. Obviously, there's no way to get scientific evidence of this, but I have observed it so often in clients, and felt it so often myself, that it simply makes more sense for me to believe than to doubt.

I don't know what part of us stores the code for our right lives—maybe some corner of the brain, maybe the figurative heart, maybe that indefinable phantasm called the soul—but I do know how the code is relayed to our conscious minds, enabling us to make choices in keeping with our purpose. It happens through the medium of the sensation we call desire. The knowledge of your destiny is available to you, well before it actually happens, as a message streaming continuously from your heart to your brain, written in the language of longing. This part of the Joy Diet is meant to help you access and interpret the yearning that is always leading you toward your right life.

Banished Desire

Menu Item #3 requires that, each day, you identify, articulate, and explore at least one thing you really want. Sounds easy enough, doesn't it? Birds do it, bees do it, even educated fleas do it—hell, even completely *un*educated fleas do it. Any sentient being knows when it wants to eat, mate, run, sleep, or fight—any sentient being, that is, except most members of the human race. We are the only beasts in creation who systematically eradicate the knowledge of our own desires.

The uniquely human ability to think abstractly and hypothesize about the future is probably to blame. At some point in all our lives—usually early on—we learn from a combination of observation, advice, and painful experience that wanting is an appallingly dangerous activity. Even as small children, we watch our elders shrink from their desires, and make mental notes to follow their example. When we don't get everything we want, the sting of unmet need conditions us against hoping again. If we dare voice a dream, we're liable to hear a litany of reasons we can't or shouldn't dream it. By the time we're adolescents, many of us have replaced the awareness of our own desires with meditations on the topic "Why I shouldn't want what I want." Crushing rebukes reverberate through our brains over and over, like endless loops in a computer program, every time we feel a desire coming on: "I'll never get what I want, so thinking about it would just frustrate me." "Desire is wicked, and I'm bad for feeling it." "If I never want anything, I'll never be disappointed." "Wanting what I want is pure selfishness."

We repeat these claims to ourselves, over and over, because we think this will allow us to avoid pain—the pain of being rebuked by others, of failure, of humiliation, of loss. One of my friends calls this self-imposed pessimism "inoculating yourself against disappointment." This is a fabulous idea, except that it doesn't work. Injecting yourself with the fruits of failure doesn't keep you well, it just makes you sick. It will stop you from doing anything that might make your dreams come true, and if something good happens to you anyway, it will keep you from enjoying or appreciating your good fortune.

Ironically, we banish most utterly those desires that are most crucial to our happiness. Did you ever notice how many award-winning children's books and films focus on someone who adopts a wild animal, then has to chase it away so that it can live normally with its own kind? The climactic scene always seems to involve the tear-drenched pet owner screaming and shaking firearms at the beloved deer or bear or snail or whatever it is, trying to make the confused creature run away and mistrust humans for the rest of its life. I think this is such a popular theme in juvenile literature because it is an archetype of the way growing humans learn to force away their desires. To handle what we think are the grim realities of life, we master the art of breaking our own hearts, then hardening what remains the way we'd put a rigid cast on a broken ankle. The more we love what we think we cannot have, the more cruelly we force it away.

This is why most of the time I spend with clients isn't devoted to helping them get what they want. That little issue is insignificant compared with the daunting task of helping them *identify* what they want. To do this, they must reexamine their deeply internalized belief that wanting is selfish or hopeless—in fact, those who don't know or respect their own wants have no foundation from which to offer generosity and compassion to others. I can't count the number of hours I've spent looking into the hollow eyes of people who are outwardly very successful, but for whom the spark of genuine desire has been either hidden or extinguished. Their resistance to becoming aware of their own wants—one of the very things that allows them to succeed in all sorts of difficult endeavors—has become so complete that it blocks access to a sense of purpose, excitement, motivation, even hope. I can tell you from extensive observation that refusing to feel desire is the only thing more painful than failing to get what you want, and that learning not to yearn, far from preventing disappointment, ultimately guarantees it.

The Danger of Desirelessness

When I suggest to clients that they explore the question "What do I want?" many of them react as though I've just offered them a hit of crack cocaine. They're shocked by the very suggestion, not because they've never thought about it, but because roiling just beneath the blank surface of their supposedly desire-less lives is a terrible dread of what might happen if they let themselves want what they want. Desire, they tell me, is a dark force, one that must be banked like the very fires of hell if it is not to consume them and everything they love.

This fear is most potent for people who are most repressed, such as those (like yours truly) who were raised in a strongly religious environment. Most Western religions have strict rules distinguishing righteous desires from evil ones, and just think-ing about something that lies outside the bounds of propriety is often considered sinful—let's not even talk about actually *wanting* such a thing. Adherents to Eastern religions also get skittish about desire, because of the premise that attachment to desire is the cause of suffering. Stop wanting, says the simplistic interpretation of these traditions, and you'll stop hurting.

This equation of desire with punishment and pain is understandable but misguided. It doesn't do justice to the key role desire plays in the very same traditions we may think are telling us to resist it. Consider the Buddhist story in which an acolyte asks his guru how to achieve enlightenment. The mas-ter responds by shoving the young man's head under water for two or three minutes, then pulling him out and saying, "When you want enlightenment as much as you just wanted air, you'll get it." The Islamic poet Kabir wrote, "When we invite the Guest into our lives, it is the intensity of the longing for the Guest that does all the work." Jesus seems to have been talking about the same kind of longing when he stated, "Blessed are they which do hunger and thirst after righteousness, for they shall be filled." Aching, longing, hungering, and thirsting are the signals by which our authentic selves call us toward our destiny. To eradicate our awareness of these sensations is to lose our place in the universe.

"But," some of my clients protest, "what if I want to do something bad? What if I want to cheat on my wife, kill my boss, drink myself to death?" I have two responses to this question.

Response #1: Your True Heart's Desires Are Never Destructive

Carl Jung said that every neurosis is a substitute for legitimate suffering. By the same token, I believe that every destructive or "bad" desire is a substitute for the constructive longing of the true self. I came to think this after spending several years doing research on addiction, interviewing scores of people who were hooked on everything from drugs to stealing to reckless anonymous sex. One day, while reading through my notes, I suddenly realized that every single person I'd interviewed was using his or her particular habit as a substitute for good emotional health, specifically the ability to give and receive love. Though these addicts' ways of trying to fulfill their desires were extremely dysfunctional, their real desires were not only natural, but essential.

My belief in the basic goodness of our deepest desires has only been reinforced during the years I've spent life-coaching hundreds of people from all walks of life. Like the addicts I interviewed, many of my clients express longings that seem destructive at first glance, but turn out to be distortions of healthy desires. For example, Tim had an obsessive craving to beat the crap out of a cousin who had bullied him throughout childhood. This desire was so graphic, so filled with hate, that I felt very nervous encouraging Tim to explore it. Nevertheless, we continued to do so for several bloodthirsty sessions, and then—just when I was wondering whether to casually mention his name to the police—Tim's wanting took an unexpected turn. From what felt like the core of his rage burst an even deeper desire: He wanted to become a child psychologist, so that he could comfort and teach children who had been victims of family violence. The moment he identified this goal, it became the driving force behind all his behavior. His lust for vengeance dried up and dropped away like an old scab. All along, Tim's bloodlust had been only the demon-mask worn by his longing to heal himself, his family, and other frightened children.

Response #2: Repressing Your Heart's Desire Leads to Destructive Action

If you believe that never letting your "bad" desires into consciousness will keep you from acting on them, or make them go away, think again. People are much more likely to act out destructive desires if they never acknowledge their feelings than if they think through them calmly and thoroughly. My friendly neighborhood addicts taught me, over and over, that the way to perpetuate an addiction is to pretend you don't want your drug. The beginning of freedom is to acknowledge that you're hooked, that you want that "bad" thing desperately. The failure to do this is exactly what leads to a Dr. Jekyll/Mr. Hyde pattern of denial, increasing tension, and desperate, damaging release. "Wanting something that's bad for you is like having a tiger loose on your property," one addict told me. "If you try to handle the situation by pretending there is no tiger, by refusing to look at it, it's sure to jump out and get you sooner or later. If you want to make sure it never hurts anyone, you have to study it until you know what makes it tick. Then you can manage it."

I have found this to be true of all messy or volatile desires. Acknowledging, articulating, and learning about them makes them manageable; denying or avoiding them gives them the power to overwhelm your best intentions. This means that Menu Item #3 is not an indulgent way to gratify your illicit longing, but an indispensable step toward living the most ethical and moral life you possibly can.

How to Want What You Want

Since most of us learn to repress our wants, the pattern of holding back, then losing control, then holding back some more, might be familiar to you. Its alternative—examining any and every one of your desires with a welcoming and curious mind—is something you may never have done. Use the instructions from Menu Item #3 to get started on this fascinating activity; you'll see how enlightening your wants can be. Continue this practice every day over weeks, months, and years, and you'll end up following the instructions that allow you to build your best destiny.

Desire-Defining Step 1: Establish a Context of Stillness

Notice that the Joy Diet doesn't ask you to rush out and grab everything you want, right now. It requires that you *identify, articulate, and explore* your heart's desires. At this point, it's imperative that you do so in the context of stillness, at least until you're sure you're sensing and acknowledging the absolute truth. Begin Menu Item #3, then, by establishing the context of "nothingness" that has become familiar to you through practicing Menu Item #1. Go to the quiet center of your awareness while you're sitting at your desk, driving to work, washing the dishes, walking the dog. But now, instead of simply being in your place of peace, begin feeling around in your heart for a sense of your desires.

It often helps to ask yourself, silently, out loud, or in writing, "What do I want most right now?" Sometimes, the answer will pop up instantly. At other times, a desire may appear as only the vaguest, most inchoate sense of yearning. Simply remain in stillness and pay attention to that feeling, without trying to force it into focus. Your heart may be telling you about a desire you're afraid to see, or something you don't even know exists. Give it time to tell its story.

For example, Alan, a manager who hated his job, was so unclear about his desires that it took me weeks to learn he loved cars—had pictures of them up all over his house, gravitated toward automotive magazines, collected Hot Wheels. As he told me this, Alan mused that his real desire might be to have a Porsche. He test-drove a couple of them but realized that buying one would still leave him wanting. His desire was bigger than that—he yearned to be around lots of different kinds of racecars. Alan began to hang out at a nearby track, but that didn't feel quite satisfying, either—he found himself yearning to *touch* the cars. When he let himself do this, the recognition of his real desire suddenly burst upon him like fireworks. What he loved about cars was that they were made of shaped metal. Alan's true self was a sculptor, with an intense drive to create fascinating, beautiful, and functional shapes out of steel. I believe he'd repressed this yearning because it didn't seem macho enough to qualify as a Manly Occupation. The last time I saw Alan, he had started his own design business, crafting gorgeous and original furniture, creating more artistic metal sculptures in his spare time, and feeling alive for the first time in years.

I spend a lot of time with clients helping them go through this process, encouraging them to grope toward the expression of desires that aren't yet on the radar screen of things they expect. I've watched doctors figure out that they want to be artists, invalids become athletes, and curmudgeons blossom into fonts of affection, all to their own surprise. I'm astonished by how often simply waiting in stillness for a desire to reveal itself leads to my clients' getting exactly what they want, even when they don't even know that their objectives exist outside the ephemeral sphere of a half-named hope.

Desire-Defining Step 2: Get Honest

Along with stillness, developing the habit of absolute honesty (something you'll have done by practicing Menu Item #2) is essential to the process of articulating desire. Knowing the feeling of a bone-deep truth is important because, no matter how well-meaning you may be, you'll almost certainly begin Menu Item #3 by lying to yourself. Why? Because some of the most rigid rules in your internal world are the ones telling you that you shouldn't want what you want. At first, you'll probably only acknowledge longings that you think are feasible, logical, and politically correct. You'll go for beauty-queen-contestant desires: peace on earth, goodwill toward men, help for the homeless, the well-being of children, and so on.

There's nothing wrong with these desires, and they can certainly be real, but unless they fill you with a sense of unbridled passion, you should follow up on them by looking for something with more emotional weight, something that makes you feel outright, pulse-pounding, grab-you-by-the-guts yearning. All of us walk around with wants we think are visceral, selfish, and inappropriate, but these are the very forbidden longings that we must understand if we are ever to overcome the obstacles to our destinies. Letting yourself do this—acknowledge with your conscious mind what your heart really, *really* wants—is similar to exposing your naked body in public: Even if you happen to be perfect, it will still make you feel very vulnerable, and if you have anything at all to hide, it requires boldness bordering on insanity. When you first start practicing Menu Item #3, wrath, gluttony, greed, and all the other Deadly Sins may come snarling and slobbering out of various subterranean cavities of your mind. Let them. Watch them. Name them. Tell the truth without flinching, and for now, do nothing else.

Desire-Defining Step 3: Pick a Pebble, Any Pebble

The yearning that spells out our destiny rarely comes into our hearts as a complete monolithic entity. Most of the time, when you go in search of your desires, you'll find them arrayed in long, loosely connected trails, like the line of white pebbles Hansel and Gretel used to find their way back from the dark forest. The longing for one specific thing leads to another, then another, then another—and then one day, quite unexpectedly, you'll realize that you are coming out of the woods into a life you love. Any little desire, so long as you truly feel it, will get you started on the path toward your destiny.

For example, the other day I asked my client Amanda to name something she wanted—anything at all. With an embarrassed laugh, she admitted that only one thing came to her mind: She wished her husband would change his hairstyle. Amanda thought this was shallow and ridiculous, but when she sat still with her desire long enough to watch it evolve, she realized that it had little to do with her husband's looks. She was changing her way of life, becoming more artistic and bohemian, and the hairstyle issue was her true self's way of saying that she hoped her husband would resurrect the "wild child" aspects of his own personality. Amanda's "shallow" desire allowed her to articulate a whole set of ideas and feelings about what her life and her marriage were meant to become. The same thing may happen when you articulate your desire for a new set of golf clubs, a walk in the park, or a really good bowl of onion soup. Don't worry how strange or trivial any given desire may seem. Focus only on whether or not it's something you truly want.

If you happen to stumble across more than one pebble at a time—in other words, if poking around in your psyche reveals several simultaneous desires—you should pick up the pebble you want most. Weigh each alternative in your mind. Which one tugs most intensely at your gut? Which seems most exciting? That's the trail you should follow. You may find that one desire calls your name over and over, every time you do this exercise, or you may have so many desires that you pick up a new one every day. That's fine. Just explore today's strongest desire, then let it go. If it pops up again tomorrow, work with it again. If something new occurs to you every single day, just follow each bit of longing to its source. You don't have to fulfill each and every desire before you go on to the next, and you can let go of a desire for years (to make room for more immediate longing) without scuttling your chances of seeing it fulfilled. Go where the love takes you, every day.

Desire-Defining Step 4: Explore Until You Find the True Desire

Like Amanda or Tim (the man who wanted to pummel his cousin), you may have initial impulses that aren't so much keys to your future as clues meant to lead you to a more profound and authentic desire. That's why, whatever your answer to the question "What do I want?" may be, you should spend some time letting the sweet ache of longing become familiar to you.

Let it grow until it feels enormous, then roam around in it, like a puppy investigating an unfamiliar backyard, exploring without judgment or inhibition. What does it really feel like, this want of yours? What are its shape and texture? What are its limits, its boundaries, its high and low points? If, for example, your knee-jerk response to the question "What do I want?" is "I want to be famous," don't back away from it. Instead, investigate. What is it about fame that you'd enjoy—being recognized on the street? Meeting other famous people? Proving to your parents that you really are important? Would you be happiest as a famous entertainer, politico, athlete, socialite, tycoon? Exactly what rewards would really fulfill your wishes?

You'll find that as you explore, your desire will expand, contract, change, evolve, ebb, and flow before settling into its true form. Gradually, you'll feel yourself reacting most intensely to the aspects of your objective that are your true heart's desires, and releasing aspects that don't match the template of your destiny. This is the sense of a true desire beginning to distinguish itself from something less authentic. Get used to it. It will save you enormous grief to experience this process mentally, as opposed to playing it out in the real world.

Possibly because of our discomfort with desire in general, most people are at least somewhat confused about how to distinguish their true desires from unhealthy impulses. An alcoholic whose true desire is to love and be loved, for example, will first feel this longing as "I want a drink," even though experience has proven that the effects of drinking are devastating. It takes focus, practice, and sometimes experimentation to tell true desires from false ones, but if you continue to study your feelings, the process gets to be as easy as telling salt from sugar. Though they may look similar at first glance, true and false desires "taste" completely different. To put it briefly, false desires taste of fear; true desires always taste of love. The emotions that underlie your wants, the logic you use to defend them, your goals in obtaining them, and the results you'll get from them are all redolent of these two different categories of emotion. If you're not sure whether you've yet arrived at the real instructions for your destiny, hold a desire in your mind and check to see whether it is best described in column 1 or column 2 of the following chart.

	FALSE DESIRES	TRUE DESIRES
FEELING:	Anxious	Joyful
	Grasping	Releasing
	Withholding	Generous
LOGICAL BASIS:	One's success means another's failure	Everyone can succeed
	Good things are scarce	Good things are abundant
	Life is about competition	Life is about cooperation
GOAL:	To impress others	To express the self
	To eliminate risk	To eliminate regret
	To control self and others	To free self and others
MEANS:	Deception	Honesty
	Secrecy	Openness
	Demand for conformity	Invitation to be unique
AFTER-EFFECTS:	Sense of hollowness	Sense of fulfillment
	Narrowing obsession	Expanding interests
	Increasing despair	Increasing inner peace

Now, mind you, there's nothing wrong with having false desires, it's just that fulfilling them at face value won't make you happy. In fact, it will diminish your happiness over the long run. If you gratify a false want over and over, ignoring the terrible feelings that accompany it, you'll move far away from your destiny and into the worst kind of despair. But the false desire itself is not evil; it is simply the lost and wandering child of some true desire. If you acknowledge and examine it with patience and compassion (though not necessarily obedience), it will lead you toward your destiny as surely as any authentic yearning.

Desire-Defining Step 5: Let Desire Become Intention

If you make Menu Item #3 a habit—in other words, if you spend some time each day paying kind attention to your desires—you will sooner or later experience something almost magical: the moment when your mind, led by your sense of yearning, embraces the next step toward the best life you are capable of living. This is the moment when desire stops being just a story about what might happen and becomes a template of what will happen; the moment when "I wish" becomes "I will."

It's difficult to describe this sensation if you've never experienced it. Sometimes, for me, it's almost a visual image, like a camera coming into focus. Many people feel it as a jolt of exhilarating energy, accompanied by just enough fear to quicken the pulse and sharpen the senses. You may feel it at the moment when you realize that you've fallen in love, or when your horrible boss starts nagging you and you realize you're about to quit, or when a casual daydream about traveling overseas suddenly becomes a plan to buy tickets. It's the realization that you not only want things you never really expected, but are about to put every ounce of your energy and will into getting them.

Quickening is an old-fashioned word that describes the moment when an expectant mother first feels her unborn child move inside her body. This is an apt metaphor for the moment desire becomes intention, because it captures the truth that although our wants come from within us, we aren't really in control of them. They have lives of their own, agendas that are largely unavailable to our conscious minds. All we can do is wait, wonder, and cherish the internal nudging that tells us something new and wonderful is preparing to be born.

Desire-Defining Step 6: Leave the Beaten Path

Once your mind is committed to fulfilling the desire coming from your heart, it will have a tendency to begin subverting the process in its own predictable, cerebral little way. It will begin looking for well-beaten paths, or better yet, well-traveled highways, that will take you to your dreams without doing anything unorthodox or difficult. For example, if you identify a burning desire to write a novel, your mind may instantly decide that you must quit your present job and move to a garret in Paris. Upon acknowledging that you are terribly lonely, your mind may conclude that you're supposed to marry the person you've been dating, even though the relationship isn't satisfying. If you want lots of money, you may assume that you have to do a job you hate in a "safe" industry, where logical people go to earn big bucks.

Your job is to check each of your mind's conclusions and suggestions for authenticity, by noticing whether they, like the original desire, spark that sense of "quickening" in your gut. If not, you are probably playing out your assumptions about what is necessary to get what you want—and this is very, very different from following the pebble-path of longing. Letting yourself be led into one heart's desire, then another, may indeed take you straight down the road you always thought you'd travel, but it may also send you off across territory no one—least of all you—ever expected you to travel. Follow your sense of yearning either way. No course of action, even the most impressively constructed and widely recommended, can lead you home if it isn't the path your soul wants to travel.

Desire-Defining Step 7: Ask "Then What?"

Your mind will also try to pigeonhole your desires into "happily ever after" events, the kinds of big achievements or victories depicted in the final scenes of romantic comedies or action-adventure films. You'll imagine yourself achieving inner peace and lifelong contentment once you graduate from Harvard, or have a baby, or reach your goal weight, or whatever. I'm using these examples because each one was a treasured fantasy of my own, at different times in my life. When I finally got them, I was crestfallen to discover that they didn't change my life the way I'd expected. In fact, my routine stayed pretty much identical. The day after I got my Harvard undergraduate degree, I started working on graduate school. The day after I had a baby, I still had to cope with all my old problems, along with about five million new responsibilities. The day I achieved my goal weight, I still had to eat right and exercise.

Sometimes, the events we think will deliver "happily ever after" actually end up making our lives worse. Say yes to people you dislike, and they'll call you more often, with higher hopes. Give your heart and soul to work you hate, and you'll end up getting promoted, so that you can do more of it. You'll be following the wrong pebble-path, to the wrong destination.

The way to avoid this is to subject your happily-ever-after image to the question "And then what?" I am known for persecuting my clients with this question.

"I want to win the lottery," a client will say (they all say this at some point).

"Okay, fine," I answer. "Then what?"

"Then I'd quit my job and move to Florida."

"Then what?"

"I'd just lie on the beach in the sun."

"Then what?"

"Then I'd just keep lying there."

"Then what?"

Though many people would genuinely enjoy a couple of weeks of beach living, I've never had a client who was truly enraptured by the thought of just sitting in the sand for the rest of eternity. Exhausted, disillusioned people need rest, but they also know they are meant to *do* something—to engage their energy and intelligence, to connect with others, to somehow make the world a better place.

You can recognize the activities that will take you toward your destiny when your answer to the question "Then what?" feels just as sweet—often even sweeter—than the fantasy of the One Great Event. The thrill of consummating a romantic attraction will be just a preface to the joy of getting up every morning, brushing your teeth, feeding the cat, and eating cereal with the person you love. The adrenaline high of performing a concert won't be any more compelling than the thought of practicing your music, hour after hour after hour. The excitement of making the team will just be a preface to the daily pleasure of working out, playing the game, getting lost in the zone of disciplined action. If your desire passes the "and then what?" test, you can be sure your mind and heart are acting in harmony.

Believe It

Once you have identified, acknowledged, and explored a true desire, you are finished with Menu Item #3 for the day. Without any further conscious effort, you will find that the desire automatically becomes central to your thinking. Your longing for this part of your right life will creep into the spaces between phone calls at work, drift through your mind as you mow the lawn, pop up in the lyrics of a song you hear on the radio. It's as though that wild animal you loved, but dutifully chased away, keeps finding its way home and crawling through every door and window of your life. You can spend the rest of your days forcing it to leave again and again and again, or you can give in to what your heart has been telling you all along: that true love—any true love, no matter how impractical, improbable, or inconvenient—is not just one of the things around which to build your right life. It's the only thing.

Believing this, after living in the school of hard knocks where we all grow up, is like thawing a frozen limb. It hurts enough to make you scream, all that once-numbed desire coming back to life, and it makes you whole again. It puts you right back where you started as a child, full of all the hope, enthusiasm, wonder, and vulnerability you thought you'd outgrown. Menu Item #3 makes you tender, in every sense of that word; open to great pain, but also to great happiness. Live with this tenderness for a while, and you cannot help changing. You'll inevitably move on toward a fresh new life—not to mention the next item on the Joy Diet.

MENU ITEM #3: DESIRE
MINIMUM DAILY REQUIREMENTS

1. Establish a context of stillness. If you have trouble stilling your inner world, practice Menu Item #1 until it begins to come easily.

2. Get honest. Ditto, Menu Item #2.

3. Pick a pebble, any pebble. Grab the first genuine desire that comes into your mind, no matter how trivial or grandiose it may seem.

4. Explore until you find the true desire. If the desire you've targeted isn't accompanied by feelings of openness, peace, and expanding interests, it isn't your core desire. Follow the trail of your desires to find the authentic yearning.

5. Let desire become intention. Begin to think of yourself as someone who doesn't just want what you want, but is going to get it.

6. Leave the beaten path. Don't assume that you will obtain the object of your desires through "normal" means; keep your mind open for unorthodox solutions.

7. Ask "Then what?" Imagine what your life will be like when your desire is fulfilled. If what follows is as satisfying as the goal itself, you've got a winner.

8. Believe that you can form your life around the fulfillment of your desires. You may have to reassure yourself when the antidesire squad starts up in your brain. Just keep telling yourself that getting what your heart really desires is possible and necessary. Eventually, experience will teach you that it's true.

CREATIVITY

•

EVERY DAY, CONCEPTUALIZE AND WRITE DOWN AT LEAST ONE NEW, CONCRETE IDEA THAT WILL HELP YOU OBTAIN SOMETHING YOUR HEART DESIRES.

"NOW," CROONS THE TEACHER OF THE YOGA CLASS I have just begun taking, "to deepen your practice, breathe into your hips and *expand* the space in your pelvis, moving your brain pan *up* toward the ceiling and your spleen *down* toward the center of the earth." Soothing sitar music plays as she demonstrates, one leg wrapped around her neck, the other folded into her armpit, her head (as far as I can tell) resting gently on the floor beside her buttocks. She looks like the very serene victim of a terrible, terrible crime. I could no more assume that position than I could fly to Neptune. Nevertheless, I am pleased to be here. This lovely woman with the buttery voice has trained her body to be so flexible and responsive that it can adapt to almost any stress placed on it, and I want to be like her.

I remember reading about an NFL receiver who studies yoga so that his limber limbs won't be surprised when they're slammed into strange positions as he plays his full-contact sport. Well, in case you haven't noticed, life is a full-contact sport, at least for the soul. One psychological equivalent of yoga, an activity that stretches and strengthens in a gentle but insistent way, is the act of creation. I'm using this term to refer to the process of realizing—making real—events, objects, or relationships that originally exist only in our imaginations. The mental image I'd like you to realize is the satisfaction of your heart's desires. If practicing Menu Item #3 has revealed that you want a life filled with travel, Menu Item #4 requires that you think of concrete ideas for building such a life. If you want inner peace, or tons of money, or a mentor, you have to come up with ideas for getting those things.

If you have a pressing desire that eclipses all others every day, Menu Item #4 will push you straight toward fulfilling it. For example, one of my clients was an elite swimmer whose passion to win an Olympic medal pushed her to the pool, burning with desire, every day. On the other hand, you may have a variety of wants that crop up on different days; on Thursday your most pressing desire is to write your novel, on Friday you want more than anything to be with a loved one. To practice Menu Item #4, just work on whatever you want most right now. If a desire continues to be important to you, it will roll around enough times, and you'll come up with enough creative ideas, to see it through. Or you'll eventually become involved with external systems that will create some other path for you and require you to work hard, whether you feel like it or not (if you want to be a doctor, you'll have to go to medical school; if you want to have a baby, you'll have to raise the little nipper even when you don't feel parental). In that case, what was once the fulfillment of Menu Item #4 has become something different. You'll learn how to handle it when we get to Menu Item #7, on play. Menu Item #4 is meant to get the ball rolling toward the satisfaction of desire. It will continue to roll if the desire is strong enough to come up repeatedly. If not, it will at least allow you to explore your own wants enough to see if you have real, sustainable passion for them.

The only way to do this is to take strange, counterintuitive positions with your mind, the way yogis do with their bodies. In the process, you'll improve your capacity to cope with all problems, from the mundane drudgeries of life, to glorious quandaries like how to love well, to big ugly dilemmas like fighting terrorism. Menu Item #4 of the Joy Diet is designed to help you become more proficient at this whole spectrum of activity. Don't worry about how stupid, impractical, grandiose, or pathetic your idea *du jour* may seem. The only thing that matters is simply that you think it up, then write it down. Every day.

Divine Discomfort

When I ask clients how they plan to get whatever they want, the typical response is bafflement tinged (sometimes more than tinged) with anger. Wait just a doggone minute, the clients fuss, aren't they paying me to solve that problem? Well, no, actually they're paying me to force *them* to solve it. If I did their mental yoga poses for them, they'd end up as inflexible and stuck as they began. This response helps me fulfill one of my own heart's desires—getting paid for doing virtually nothing—but it also happens to be true. My clients don't like it, though, because creation requires a stretching of the mind that can be so uncomfortable many people spend their whole lives avoiding it.

As you start on Menu Item #4, you should know that it may cause persistent psychological discomfort, and that this is a good thing. In yoga, they call this "going to your edge," moving into a position where you feel *slightly* uncomfortable, and staying right there as your range of motion slowly increases. Going past your edge, in contrast, causes outright pain, which will condition you to avoid it, which will actually make you less flexible. Once you know how it feels to go to the edge of your creative capacity, you'll begin to see that problems are solved by leaning into this sensation, not retracting from it. On many days, Menu Item #4 will be a challenge. Accepting that challenge as part of the process will allow you to stop getting in the way of your own creativity. Here are some uncomfortable truths you might as well know, right at the outset.

Uncomfortable Truth #1: You Are Always Responsible for Creating Your Life, Whether You Like It or Not

It's unfortunate that the word *creativity* is most often associated either with great art or the sort of finger-painting courses you might take down at the community center if you had a lot of free time and a mild mental illness. Most people fall in between these two sides of the spectrum, and these folks are accustomed to thinking that they are not creating anything. I say that belief is weasel waste. Even if you never go near the arts, you are creating away like mad every single day, working in the medium of experience itself. Actions, objects, words, gestures— literally anything you influence by your choices becomes part of your creation. Every time you voice your thoughts to a loved one, or cook a meal, or choose a new bar of soap for the dish by your bathtub, you are creating a modification in space or time that would never have existed without you. Whether consciously or unconsciously, you have more power to create your own life than anyone or anything else.

This can be hard to swallow if you're in difficult or disappointing circumstances. For example, Christine came to me after failing at a series of jobs and relationships. Smart, hardworking, and well-intentioned, Christine had no idea why everything always went wrong for her just when it looked as though she was about to succeed. After a few minutes of poking around in her psyche, Christine and I discovered one of those good-news, bad-news truths. First, the bad news: Christine had a very powerful belief, taught to her (unconsciously) by her parents, that she should do well in life, but never quite so well that she'd become free of her dependency on them. Now the good news: Christine hadn't been failing at all—in fact, she always succeeded in doing exactly what she set out to do: achieving early success in every endeavor, then self-sabotaging at the very moment when she was about to reach financial and emotional independence. What Christine had taken to be inexplicable bad luck or a demonstration of helplessness was actually an expression of her power as a creator.

Understanding that you have this kind of power can be painful and disgruntling, because it requires that you accept responsibility for much of your past, present, and future experience—no shifting the blame, no playing the victim, no passing the buck. If you don't like this, please allow me to suggest (in the kindest, most supportive way) that you suck it up and deal. It's well worth owning your role in imperfect creations if it means embracing the full, breathtaking extent of your creative power.

Uncomfortable Truth #2: Creation Is Hard

"My wife plays the violin really well," a client named Benjamin told me, "but she's not talented. She just works hard."

With this one offhand comment, Benjamin explained his fifty years of dogged underachievement. Aha, I remember thinking. Here is one of those artistically ambitious people who believe that talent means success without effort. Benjamin had been searching vainly for his own genius all his life, because he didn't know what it would look like. He thought he'd recognize it by the magnificent work that would spill out of him spontaneously, perhaps while he was napping. He never expected talent to come wrapped in the slow, messy, awkward, humbling work every creator will sooner or later have to face. Michelangelo once said, "If people knew how hard I work, they wouldn't find my achievements so remarkable." Like Benjamin, most people attribute creative achievement to great ease, when in fact it comes from great effort.

People with Benjamin's mind-set tend to be very—sometimes viciously—critical. Their assumption that creation is easy not only stops them in their tracks the moment they encounter any difficulty, but makes them feel justified in lambasting other people for the way they raise their children, do their jobs, live their lives. Criticism is an alluring substitute for creation, because tearing things down, unlike building them up, really is as easy as falling off a stump. It's blissfully simple to strike a savvy, sophisticated pose by attacking someone else's creations, but the old adage is right: Any fool can burn down a barn. Building one is something else again.

To go to the edge of your creativity means that you constantly challenge yourself to stay in the trenches, to solve and build and make, rather than waiting for effortless success or tearing other people's work apart. When you look at the work of a creative master, don't assume that it was easy; study it to see how the genius worked, and remind yourself that with an enormous amount of effort, you might learn to work the same way.

Before you make negative comments about other people's creations, require yourself to do a better job than they did, under similar conditions. Remember that you, like anyone else, can only realize the grand vision in your mind's eye by working with the grubby, recalcitrant tools of the material world.

Uncomfortable Truth #3: Creation Usually Doesn't Work

A friend of mine once called, with gloomy triumph in his voice, to read me the results of a study showing that pessimists are right more often than optimists. I was not surprised. Because creation is difficult and problematic, even the best-laid plans really do go awry. Whether you set out to make a fortune, or a friendship, or a positive difference in the lives of zoo animals, your chance of succeeding at any given attempt is much smaller than your chance of failing. Being an optimist myself (and therefore usually wrong, but not about this), I don't believe the daunting odds mean we should stop trying to create lives filled with joy. I think it means we should try more often, in more ways.

In my life-coaching work, I've noticed that the biggest difference between wildly successful people and total failures is that the successful people fail more. They throw their hearts into one hopeful venture after another, and most of these efforts fall flat. Comedy writer John Vorhaus claims that the failure rate in his profession is about 90 percent. He calls this the "Rule of Nine," meaning that for every good joke a comic writes, there will be nine more that are about as funny as leprosy. Successful comedians aren't necessarily people who hit the funny bone 100 percent—or even 50 percent—of the time. They're just people who write a thousand jokes, then drop the nine hundred that don't work.

I encourage you to remember the Rule of Nine when you set out to create ideas for fulfilling your desires. I also suggest that you have the following statement (which I have said before and will repeat until my last breath) tattooed on a highly visible patch of your skin:

IF SOMETHING IS WORTH DOING, IT'S WORTH DOING BADLY.

This is the basic premise that helps all successful creators keep trying in the face of frequent failure. On any given day, the creative ideas you think up for Menu Item #4 will be terrible. Well done! You're one bad idea closer to a good one.

Thinking It Up, Writing It Down

Now that you know some of the ugly truths about developing creative ideas, let's get down to the actual process. Actually, if you've been practicing the first three elements of the Joy Diet on a regular basis, you've already completed the most important part. Accurately and specifically stating the question to be answered, the desire to be fulfilled, ensures that your creative ideas will address the right problem. Most people who aren't consciously building their lives never get this far. Their plans for living come from half-formed inclinations and other people's demands, meaning that their creativity is never targeted at resolving the issues that really matter to them. So take your time with Menu Items #1, #2, and #3 before you plunge into creation.

When you're ready for Menu Item #4, you'll need a piece of paper and a writing instrument. Start by writing down your desire in the form of a "how" question. For example, if your desire is "I want to date an Army Ranger," write, "How can I get an Army Ranger to date me?" or "How might I go about dating an Army Ranger?" If your desire is "I want a new hamster," try whatever question best fits your situation. For one person, it might be "How do I afford a new hamster?" For another individual, it might be "How do I find out how to care for a hamster?" or "How can I find out where to get the breed of hamster I want?"

Now, write down at least five answers to this question. Be imaginative and open, even a little weird. The important thing here is quantity, not quality, so bully for you if your proposed solutions seem silly, embarrassing, or impossible. Letting yourself come up with wild, ridiculous ideas starts the flow of creativity, and a reasonable (but heretofore unimagined) solution may show up when you least expect it. In fact, the best way to come up with good solutions to stubborn problems is to think up strange or silly or startling things you might do to fulfill your heart's desires. As soon as you come up with just one answer that might be possible, you're finished with your daily practice of Menu Item #4.

If you find yourself chewing on your pencil like a bunny rabbit with a carrot stick, unable to think of one single idea, or if you've reached the limit of your present imagination, don't think of it as a dead end. It's actually an opportunity to have a conceptual breakthrough. As Einstein said, no problem was ever solved from within the frame of thought that created the problem in the first place. Creation always involves moving beyond the limitations of your current worldview. This is where a little mental yoga can help. Listed next are some techniques designed to put your brain in unfamiliar postures. They can help you churn out so many lousy ideas that sooner or later, a good one comes along. Holding your unfulfilled desire in mind, try the following techniques.

Creativity Step 1: Force Innovation

I have a teacher friend who instructs up to a hundred students each year. She always begins her class by asking each classroom-full of students to move across a patch of floor. There's just one catch: No one is allowed to cross the distance in a way someone else has already done it. The first few students take all the obvious methods—walking backward, crawling, hopping, skipping. The next few get a little bamboozled, until suddenly, someone has a breakthrough idea—using a rolling chair, for instance, or cooperating with other students to move in various innovative ways. The more methods get used up, the more new ways occur to the children. In addition, my friend tells me that every year, someone comes up with an idea she's never seen before. Forcing yourself to think up something unprecedented opens up worlds of possibilities just when you'd expect to run out of ideas. The Joy Diet requires at least one solid, feasible new idea a day, but the truth is that if you had to, you could come up with twenty.

Creativity Step 2: Perseverate on Your Enemies

To "perseverate" is a psycho-babble term that means to mentally focus on one topic to the point of obsession. If you never perseverate about anything, you can skip this exercise—but I think that highly unlikely. Most of us have our favorite brooding subjects. We may perseverate about our loneliness, our children's behavior, the spread of Africanized killer bees, whatever. There may be a type of personality (permissive, anal-retentive, controlling) that sends us into a fury whenever we encounter it in anyone. We may focus relentlessly on one person, perseverating for decades about a current or bygone relationship.

This exercise begins with identifying one person, or group of people, about whom you often brood. I'm particularly interested in the people you absolutely cannot stand, scumbags whose behavior is so grossly reprehensible that you can spend hours thinking about how bad they are. Be honest as you name this person or group. For the moment, don't worry about sounding rational, or open-minded, or politically correct. I've spent entire months of my life perseverating about how much I loathe people who have never been anything but nice to me. I've condemned entire professions with little justification. For example, I went through a phase where I pretty much detested anyone with a Ph.D. Was this fair or right? Of course not. Did it help me figure out creative ways to get what I wanted from life? Oh yes, it did, once I began approaching it in the following way. First, write down the person or group you find particularly infuriating. This is the name of The Enemy.

NAME YOUR ENEMY

I really, really can't stand _____

Now, think about whatever it is that you hate most about your enemy. What is it about them, what do they do, that really knots your knickers? This doesn't even have to be a real trait or behavior. It might be completely fictional, a product of your jaded imagination. Go ahead and pinpoint it, whether it's justified or not.

For example, I used to believe that people with Ph.D.s were all overschooled, self-congratulatory narcissists with no experience of real life. My client Dorothy confessed to detesting women who wear revealing clothes—she saw them as oversexed and stupid. Bill hates police officers; he thinks they're dangerous, controlling bigots. Helen obsesses constantly about her mother, who, at fifty-eight, still acts as helpless as a five-year-old. What is it about your enemy that drives you nuts? Write down—honestly, now!—whatever comes to mind.

NAME YOUR ENEMY'S EVIL DEEDS

The thing that bothers me most about [your enemy's name goes here] is _____

You may well find that the space provided isn't nearly big enough to contain all the things you hate about your enemy. Fine! Go into your usual perseveration mode, then make a list of the really horrid traits your enemy displays. This may take a little time, but what the heck—it's time you'd otherwise spend brooding about this very topic. In the following space, write down the qualities of the enemy you most detest.

LIST OF ENEMY TRAITS

I especially hate the following things about my enemy:

1. _____

2. _____

3. _____

Continued

4. _____

5. _____

So far, you're probably feeling pretty good about this exercise. Perseverating on one's enemies is a very enjoyable pastime, very reinforcing to the ego. Unfortunately, that portion of the party is over. I am now going to suggest that the traits and behaviors you just listed may be *exactly* the things you should incorporate into your own behavior, in order to fulfill your heart's desires. Yes, that's right. I'm asking you to adopt all the behaviors you hate most, to join—or at least learn from—the enemy.

The rationale behind this suggestion is that we don't brood on things unless they are psychologically important to us. When the object of our obsession is another person, it's usually because that person embodies an aspect of ourselves that we are trying to incorporate and accept. This is just as true of those we hate most as it is of those we love most. It could well be that the reason your thoughts revolve around this enemy is that you're looking in a kind of mirror, one that shows you all the things you think you must not be. Judgmental, condemnatory brooding is often our way of resisting parts of ourselves that we have dispossessed because we believe them to be bad. This belief keeps us rigid, stuck in one position, unable to explore the range of our own personalities, and therefore unable to approach life creatively. This doesn't mean that your enemies are morally right, or that you shouldn't detest them. It does mean that you may need a reframed version of their characteristics in your own behavioral repertoire.

For example, my Ph.D.-hating stage came right after I'd had a mentally retarded child and moved away from Harvard, where I, myself, was a doctoral candidate. I wanted to fit in with other young mothers, and I wanted the world to accept my son regardless of his IQ scores. I was unconsciously—but very rigorously—rejecting the part of myself that actually liked hanging out with bookish, ambitious people at a prestigious university. I couldn't stop brooding about how much I hated academics, because part of me wouldn't let go of the fact that I was one, and that having a Ph.D., unfair as this may be, would help me fulfill my dreams. Until I accepted the part of me that was (how did I put it?) an overschooled, self-congratulatory narcissist with no experience of real life, I wasn't able to use the full range of my abilities and credentials to obtain my heart's desires.

Here are some examples of the way this exercise worked for the clients I mentioned earlier: Dorothy's life changed dramatically when she actually began trying on, then buying and wearing, the kind of sexy clothes she'd always condemned. It turned out that Dorothy could look pretty darn sexy herself, something she'd been taught was wicked, provocative, and likely to get her in the worst kind of trouble. It didn't. After incorporating her sexuality more fully, she had a much better marriage and a more vivid life. Bill realized that his hatred of police officers was partially his true self asking him to stop being a soft-spoken doormat. There was a tough-guy hero in Bill's sensitive soul, and embracing that fact gave him a sense of balance and self-confidence. Helen's relationship with her mother changed dramatically when Helen realized that she'd always played the grown-up in the relationship, while her mother played the child. When Helen let herself be more childish—less patient, less long-suffering, more aware of her own need to be nourished—she set better boundaries, giving her mother less resentment-filled attention and more incentive to grow up.

Reexamine the traits you listed in the preceding box, with the consciousness that they may be exactly what you need to accept in yourself. Then, approach the problem of fulfilling your desires from the perspective of the "enemy." If you hate lazy people, you may be able to solve your problems only if you're willing to stop working so hard. If you're a woman who broods about the terrible qualities of men, you may need to use strategies and personality traits you consider masculine— ditto if you're a man who can't stand women. If you are appalled by other people's sloppiness, you may be pushing away a solution to your problems because it seems messy. Think of ways you can incorporate aspects of your enemies, and you're likely to find a new perspective from which altogether new ideas emerge.

Creativity Step 3: Unify False Dichotomies

There are two groups of people in this world: those who divide people into two groups, and those who don't. Seriously, there actually is a stage of psychological development characterized by "dichotomous thinking," or believing that the universe consists of pairs of opposites. Psychologist Carl Rogers built a whole school of therapy on the premise that false dichotomies play a role in most dysfunctional behavior. When we believe that everything in our lives is "either/or," we tend to switch from one extreme position to its opposite, never exploring the infinite ways of thinking that lie in between or elsewhere altogether.

For example, Kim lived on the edge, going to wild parties and living in a garret, until she had a child and suddenly became a "good girl" who never did anything for fun. Leonard thought that becoming a doctor meant he would be married to his career, unable to sustain a fulfilling relationship. Lorraine thought that if she wanted a cat, she'd have to stay on disagreeable allergy medication. All of these people thought they had to choose between just two possible options. This kept them from seeing ways in which their problems might be solved.

To shake yourself free of falsely dichotomous thinking, try making a list of either/ors in your life. These could be any pairs of opposites, contradictory things that you could be, have, or do.

MY DICHOTOMOUS LIFE

I can either be _____ or _____

I can either have _____ or _____

I can either do _____ or _____

Now, rewrite those very same things in the box below:

MY CREATIVE LIFE

I intend to be both _____ and _____

I intend to have both _____ and _____

I intend to do both _____ and _____

Initially, you'll feel a lot of resistance to what you've written in the box "My Creative Life." The more angry it makes you ("No, dammit, I can*not* be both a professional hula dancer and a Supreme Court Justice!"), the more likely it is that the dichotomy comes from false ideas, rather than reality. Even if they upset you, *especially* if they upset you, say or write the sentences in that box several times. Notice that each repetition creates a small change in the way you feel. Your rigidity may begin to wiggle, the way your baby teeth did before they fell out. By stating something you thought impossible, you have set your mind in motion creating unorthodox solutions. Rejecting the word *or* and substituting *and* encourages your creative little brain to come up with ways and means it may otherwise have kept to itself.

I've seen dozens of clients come up with equally unusual ways of solving problems, using the raw materials of their lives in combinations they may never have thought possible. Kim's whole life changed when she realized that she could blend the requirements of motherhood with friendship and festivity, and that having both gave her a sense of balance she'd always lacked. Leonard set up his own medical practice to give himself autonomy, worked fewer hours than most of his colleagues, and ended up marrying another doctor who joined him as a business partner. Individually, they made less money than doctors who worked more hours, but their quality of life was much better. Lorraine preserved both her health and her love for felines when she bought a congenitally hairless cat named Pinkie, who didn't trigger her allergies. Pinkie looked to me like a large, hideous, insectoid fetus, but Lorraine adored him.

Creativity Step 4: Break the Rules of the Garden of Eden

As you may remember from this week's Bible study, the one thing Adam and Eve were supposed to do in the Garden of

Eden was to stay the hell away from the Tree of the Knowledge of Good and Evil. The thing that got them thrown out of the Garden wasn't sex or violence or failing to clean up their apple cores; it was awareness. Whether or not you believe this story literally, it metaphorically parallels the process that happens when we become aware of the unspoken dynamics at work in any social situation. For example, every family has implicit rules about the way things should work, rules that everyone keeps religiously: maybe Dad always gets his way, or everyone tiptoes around Mabel's delicate emotions, or no one mentions Kelly's divorce. Whatever the rules are, there is virtually always a crucial über-rule: *No one is allowed to talk openly and honestly about the rules.* Becoming aware of these rules means that we can no longer follow them out of habit and ignorance; having seen the way the system works, we are confronted by the possibility and responsibility of making choices.

The strategy of breaking the über-rule—talking about the rules at work in a system, rather than simply keeping those rules—works amazingly well at breaking logjams that have to do with human relationships, whether romantic, familial, friendly, or professional. One of my group-therapist friends calls this "going to the balcony," because doing it is like stepping away from whatever drama is occurring, and analyzing the drama itself, from the cheap seats. For instance (since we've been talking about my doctoral-candidate days), one of my graduate school professors was a gruff man who tended to give feedback laced with profanity and insults. One day he told me that a paper I'd turned in was "the worst f-ing thing he'd ever read." The logical reaction, which came into my head immediately, was to shoot myself. Then, since I was already as good as dead, it occurred to me to head for the balcony.

"Could I ask you a question?" I said.

"You just did, you cretin," he told me.

"True," I said, "but I'm wondering—do you really hate me, or is this just the way you teach?"

He thought for a second or two, then said, "It's just the way I teach."

From that moment on, I found this particular man far easier to work with, and weirdly enough, he started acting as though he kind of liked me.

I've coached clients through hundreds of tiny—and not so tiny—confrontations like this one. Wayne was nearly mad with anxiety trying to work with a boss who seemed determined to fire him. When he up and told the boss, "I think you're determined to fire me," he found that his boss was under the impression Wayne was trying to get *him* fired. Louise spent an anguished year wondering if the man she loved could ever love her back. When she finally raised the issue, it turned out that he'd taken her reticence as a sign not to come on so strong. Going to the balcony, articulating the rules, eating the fruit of the Tree of Knowledge; whatever you call this process, it banishes childlike ignorance and leaves us staring right at the realities of our relationships. This may be frightening, because it gives us the power of the Creator, the ability and responsibility to make up our lives as we go along. It will open the floodgates of your imagination.

Creativity Step 5: Combine the Incongruous

One of the mistakes my clients often make is focusing all their attention on things that relate to the life problem they're trying to solve. If the issue is career-related, they read dozens of career guidance books, go to career counselors, check out career-development websites. If they want to meet the perfect partner, they post their names on dating services or hang out at singles bars. If they want to become famous painting oils, they imitate brilliant oil painters. Whatever your desire, there's nothing wrong with pursuing obvious ways to fulfill it. However, the odds of succeeding will be greatly enhanced if you also do things that are as far from obvious as possible. If I had a client who was facing any or all of the problems I've just named, I'd recommend that they pursue activities like playing jazz clarinet, reading physics, or fishing. Dividing attention between the expected and the unexpected creates unusual juxtapositions of ideas, and these are fabulous for sparking innovative thinking.

You can also create incongruous ideas by talking with people who think very differently. Discuss your heart's desires with three of the most dissimilar people you can find—say, your sixth-grade teacher, your secretary, and the immigrant taxi driver who takes you home one day. Put their responses together in your mind, shake well, and see what develops. Sometimes one or more of their ideas will be good ones. At other times, the blend of differences will yield an idea that's altogether new. Most of the ideas I use in life coaching, both in person and in writing, come from combining the perspectives of Asian and Western thought, motherhood and the professional world, professional demands and intuitive impressions. The more different the perspectives I bring to bear on a problem, the more innovative and effective the solution.

Creativity Step 6: Do One Thing Different

I've borrowed the phrase "do one thing different" from Bill O'Hanlon, a psychologist who wrote a book by that title. O'Hanlon's premise is that we can get out of psychological ruts by changing one thing, anything, about our customary way of approaching the problem. For example, if a couple keeps repeating the same argument over and over, O'Hanlon might suggest that they go ahead and repeat it—only the next time they start, each of them must put on a hat, or climb into the empty bathtub, or lie on the floor. Then the argument can continue.

I've found that this technique works very well for me and my clients. Changing one part of a routine makes it extremely difficult not to notice that other things could be different, as well. Paying your bills while sitting at a café table, rather than your desk, can help you figure out how to manage your finances. Driving a new route to work can give you the idea that helps you lose that stubborn weight. How, where, and when will this occur? I have no idea. You're the one who will find out, at the moment it happens. All I know is that by putting yourself in unfamiliar situations, you'll see things with fresh eyes, and solutions you may never have noticed will crop up, one after another, until you realize that you've just had a very, very bright idea, one that might just help you realize your heart's desires. Write it down.

The Take-Away

If you went through all the preceding exercises with your desire firmly in mind, and still have no possible answers to your question, you may want to bring in extra minds, in the form of friends, loved ones, a therapist, or a life coach like me. But I've found that it's hard for my clients to actually do the exercises without having new ideas. My bet is that, by hook or by crook, you'll create yourself a nice tidy list of ideas, at least one of which will be feasible.

Now that you've got your creative idea written down, what should you do with it? Whatever you want. Post it, memorize it, forget it, burn it, file it—I don't really care. The important thing, the thing that will change your life most, is that you've learned to take a creative approach to solving your life's most important puzzles. Doing this once every day is like physical yoga; it improves your overall fitness and increases your ability to accomplish things that may seem totally unrelated to your actual exercise session. Consistently practicing Menu Item #4 will mean that you begin coming up with creative ideas all day long. Some will seem absolutely logical ("Why didn't I think of that before?") and some will seem downright bizarre ("Oh my gosh, do you think I really could . . . ?"). Either way, they'll have a resonance that will not allow you to dismiss them. You don't have to worry about hanging on to them, because they will hang on to you.

The ideas that stick in your mind are the ones you'll take into the next stage of the Joy Diet. You may want to hang on to your written list as a basis for Menu Item #5, but you don't have to. Just by writing them down, even if you do nothing else with them, you have begun the process of externalizing in tangible reality the creations of your unique imagination. Now you are ready to move into the world of action, to buckle down and put your ideas to work. I hope you're well stretched-out and limbered up, because what's coming next could be a wild ride.

MENU ITEM #4: CREATIVITY

MINIMUM DAILY REQUIREMENTS

Think it up and write it down.

Begin your daily practice by writing down your most pressing heart's desire in the form of a question ("How could I . . . ?"). Then write five possible answers. If none of them are feasible, write five more. Continue until at least one feasible idea emerges.

To increase the range of your creativity, try the following "mind-yoga" techniques.

1. Force innovation. Think of ten ways to solve the problem you're facing. These solutions don't have to be sensible, ethical, or even legal. The only thing they must be is different from each other. Got that? Good. Now think of ten more.

2. Perseverate on your enemies. Target an individual or group you hate. Say what you hate most about them. See if a reframed version of this quality might be something you either need, or already have. Let yourself act as your enemy acts, within your moral boundaries.

3. Unify false dichotomies. Make a list of things that cannot coexist in your behavior, your environment, or your life. Commit to being, doing, or having both of them. See if a solution arises.

4. Break the rules of the Garden of Eden. Begin to notice the unspoken rules of a social system you live with. Describe the dynamics you see at work in the situation. Do it right out loud.

5. Combine the incongruous. Think of a problem you have to solve in order to achieve a heart's desire. Set out to do something that has absolutely nothing to do with this problem. Allow your mind to simply observe; if it sees a solution, it will tell you.

6. Do one thing different. As you go through customary activities, change your behavior in one way. Walk a different route to the kitchen, eat spaghetti with your fingers, walk the cat.

Once you get a feasible idea about how to realize your heart's desire, do whatever you want with it. Use ideas that stick as a basis for Menu Item #5.

RISK

•

EVERY DAY, DO AT LEAST ONE FRIGHTENING THING THAT CONTRIBUTES TO THE FULFILLMENT OF YOUR DESIRES.

I AM WRITING THIS ON A PLANE BOUND FOR SAN Francisco, where my friend Isabella has just received a potentially scary medical diagnosis. The word *tumor* has been mentioned. This is especially nerve-racking because the symptoms that sent Isabella to the doctor are the same ones her mother developed on the way to a slow, excruciating death just a few years ago. Tomorrow, with her mother's ordeal still fresh in her memory, Isabella is supposed to return to her doctor for more testing.

My mind (being, after all, my mind) has immediately leapt to the worst-case scenario, so right now I'm scared on a number of levels. First and foremost, I'm afraid of what Isabella may have to endure. I'm also selfishly afraid of losing my friend to the Grim Reaper. And then there's the more prosaic, small-minded fear that I may be doing the wrong thing by going to San Francisco. See, when I asked Isabella if she'd like me to come, she said no. She's very busy at her high-pressure job—

really, she told me, if I showed up, it would just put more stress on her, something she needs like . . . well, cancer.

I was going to honor Isabella's request, I really was. The problem is that I'm on the Joy Diet, and whenever I go through the first three menu items—a few minutes of stillness, followed by a moment of truth, followed by identifying my heart's desire—I realized that what I want most today is to be available for my friend if she happens to need me. After doing Menu Item #4, I've come up with a plan that I think will meet both my needs and Isabella's: I'll fly to San Francisco, get a hotel room in her neighborhood, then stay in telephone contact without mentioning I'm in town. If she decides at the last minute that she could use some company during or after the testing procedures, I'll only be a few minutes away. If not, I'll just go home.

A large part of me sees, with radiant clarity, that this is the plan of an imbecile. I've always dreaded imposing myself where I'm not wanted, and I know I'm probably indulging a codependent need, stemming from my memory of how much I wanted company when I was undergoing medical tests myself. My present course of action might actually make things worse for Isabella, and embarrassing for me. But I'm sitting here, between a man who has fallen asleep on my shoulder and a woman who just spilled her drink perilously close to my laptop, because I am in the habit of taking risks on behalf of my heart's desires. For me, going to San Francisco is today's version of Menu Item #5. I have no idea how it will play out, but I promise to let you know before this chapter is over.

This is an unusually eventful example of Menu Item #5. Ordinarily I don't travel long distances or spend chunks of money to stay on this part of the Joy Diet. Yesterday, for example, my

Menu Item #5 activity consisted of saying "no" to a speaking invitation. (This may not sound like a biggie to you, but it sets off a cascade of people-pleasing anxiety in me.) However, as we'll see, if you add this menu item to your daily routine in small ways, you'll probably end up having large adventures. Start by thinking through the ideas you dreamed up doing Menu Item #4, and go looking for fear in any of its guises: anxiety, nervousness, uneasiness, outright terror. Work your creativity until you arrive at an idea that makes you shrink away, a little or a lot. The fear shows that you have reached the border of your personal comfort zone. You're about to push that border back and claim new territory in your own life, the only way you can: by taking risks.

Why Risk?

Almost all my clients eventually reach a point where they know what they want from life and have several creative ideas about how to make it happen. At this point, without exception, they find themselves facing some action step that scares them. It might be anything: switching jobs, confronting a psycho-neighbor, writing a book, adopting a child. Some clients go right out and grab this scary proposition by the mane and tail. Others stall . . . and stall . . . and stall. I used to think that if I could just give the really severe stallers enough support and comfort, their fears would disappear, allowing them to move forward stress-free. I was wrong. In the end, I did these people a great disservice by making their stagnation more comfortable. Some of them stayed at the very brink of crucial risks for months, even years, and never actually took them.

These days, I'm less like a nurturing, nondirective therapist than a skydiving instructor who stands at the open door of an airplane and methodically shoves terrified students into thin air. Experience has taught me that the way to a joyful life is always fraught with fear, that to find it you must follow your heart's desires right through the inevitable terrors that arise to hold you back. If you don't do this, your life will be shaped by fear, rather than love, and I guarantee, the shape will be narrow and tiny compared with your best destiny.

If you find yourself balking at the idea that risk is a must-have ingredient for a joyful life, consider the fact that living to avoid fear is more dangerous to your true self than a life full of obvious risks. It precludes all the rewards that can only come by daring to try, and it can never avert all tragedy. In *Moby-Dick,* Herman Melville described rowing a whale boat while knowing that the ropes attached to the harpoons, the "whale lines," could yank him to his death at any moment. He wrote that he didn't feel any less safe in this situation than he did sitting in his living room, because death could come anywhere. We are all surrounded by whale lines, he said, no matter where we are. Whether we are at ease or afraid depends more on our perceptions than our circumstances.

If you really put it to the test, you'll probably find that your comfort zone is arbitrary and irrational. Most people's are. You may know someone who's terrified of flying, but feels perfectly comfortable driving 80 miles per hour while simultaneously eating, talking on the phone, and shaving. The same folks who fearlessly have unprotected sex (say, to break the ice with new acquaintances) are often utterly terror-stricken at the thought of saying "I love you." There are people who carefully guard against the danger of being attacked by strangers, but who docilely return, day after day, to a home where they know they'll get beaten up by their domestic partners. These folks— like the rest of us—feel secure in situations they *believe* to be safe, even though they may be in mortal danger.

Taking risks that may help you achieve your dreams is the only way to challenge the fearful beliefs that have kept you from achieving them already. It provides empirical evidence to support or disprove your various hypotheses about how the world works. It breaks down the boundaries set by fear, and this will decimate the constraints that are keeping you from your right life. I've gotten increasingly tough about pushing clients through Menu Item #5 because, in a weird way, I've actually come to enjoy taking my own risks. The frisson of fear that runs through me as I contemplate my daily adventure sometimes precedes disaster, but just as often, it means I'm on the way to experiencing more confidence, more understanding, and more joy than I've ever felt before.

The longer I practice this menu item, the better I get at assessing which risks are worth taking, and which are just plain stupid (trust me, I've had lots of experience with the latter). I've also learned how you can make a desirable risk as safe as possible, figuratively strapping on a parachute, or at least a bungee cord, before you take your leap of faith. In the rest of this chapter, I'll tell you everything I know that might help you minimize the fear you feel as you do what it takes to create your best life. But don't worry, I can't take away the whole thrill. After reading the best advice I can offer, you'll still be scared to death. Count on it.

How to Spot a Good Risk

Contrary to conventional wisdom, a good risk is not necessarily one that leads to success. *Any risk worth taking is worth taking whether it leads to success or failure.* The criterion by which you should decide which dangers to face, and which to avoid, is not your chance of succeeding but the depth of your desire. If you pursue only risks that are interwoven with your heart-strings, your life will be what it should be, no matter what the outcome of a given situation. If your objective isn't something you really want, even a tiny risk is a stupid one.

Martin Luther King Jr. once said that no one is truly free who is afraid to die. He did exactly as his heart's desires dictated, went flat out for his famous dream—and got killed for it. Would he have taken the same risks, made such bold moves, if he'd been aware of the outcome? You know me well enough by now to guess my answer: I think he probably *was* aware of it. But he also knew that following his truth was a smaller risk than continuing to play the obedient subordinate in an unjust society. The latter option might have saved his life, but it would have destroyed his soul.

I hope you and I never face such difficult options, but the same dynamics that operate in famous martyrs' lives apply to even our humblest choices. Do we take the course of action that serves our real desires, or do we surrender ourselves, little by little, to the dictates of fear? My client Lora, a brilliant artist who recently resumed painting after years of inactivity, told me that she stood in her kitchen every New Year's Day for twenty years, washing dishes and thinking, "Next year will be different. I can't go another year without doing what I love." When she finally did start painting professionally, it felt like a huge risk, but as Lora said, "How could I possibly lose as much by trying as I did by refusing to try? What's safe about not being who you were meant to be?"

When you're wondering whether to take a certain risk, try answering the following questions.

RISK ASSESSMENT

When considering a course of action that scares you, ask yourself . . .

1. Is this risk really necessary to achieve my heart's desires? Do I feel a genuine longing for whatever it is I'm seeking?

2. Does the thought of taking this step create an inner sense of clarity, despite my apprehensions? (When a risk is good for you, you may feel apprehension, but little or no confusion.)

3. Do I feel only fear, or is there also a sense of toxicity akin to disgust? (Pay attention. A good risk feels like taking a high dive into a sparkling clean pool; a bad risk feels like taking the same leap, but into polluted swamp water.)

4. At the end of my life, which will I regret more: taking this risk and failing, or refusing to take it, and never knowing whether I would have succeeded or failed?

Answering these questions has landed me in thousands of situations that felt risky, beginning when I was fourteen (the age when I decided to do one frightening thing a day), and continuing until this very minute, on this plane to San Francisco. For every exciting success I've experienced, there have been many, many failures. But I can honestly say that I don't regret one risk I took on behalf of my real heart's desires, whether or not the outcome was what I had hoped. What regret I do feel is reserved for the times I backed away from a risk my true self was urging me to take.

How to Risk

If you have any reservations about Menu Item #5, it's probably because you're scared. I suggest that you count reading on, with an open mind, as having fulfilled this step of your daily Joy Diet regimen. Here, in detail, is the process that should become very familiar to you once you've integrated this menu item into your routine.

Risk-Taking Step 1: Choose Any Scary Goal

Begin your daily risk-taking exercise by contemplating a scary course of action you need to take in order to achieve your desires. It could be something you've written down while doing Menu Item #4, or it could be something that's always on your mind, like "Stand up to my mother when she criticizes me," or "Find some friends who really get me," or "Make more money." Specify an action step, something you could do today that would—or anyway, could—take you closer to your heart's desires.

Okay, now do it.

Wait, no, come back! That was just a simulation, to see how you responded to the challenge of acting on the plans you've devised. If you went bounding off full of enthusiasm, like a greyhound after a hare, you'll have to identify a riskier action step. If you felt yourself floundering, resisting, or hesitating, even for a moment, you've located a part of your life plan worthy of Menu Item #5. Jot it down in the following space.

ONE RISKY THING I COULD DO TO OBTAIN MY HEART'S DESIRES

_____

_____

_____

_____

_____

If you're having trouble identifying a desirable risk, try thinking of different categories of danger. Almost everyone is braver about certain types of risk than others. Some of the following probably make you nervous, even if most don't. You don't want to leap into these frightening activities helter-skelter, just to say you did it. You only have to identify which fears are keeping you from your heart's desires, even though careful thought, preparation, and caution might allow you to do them safely.

TYPES OF RISK

CATEGORY	DESCRIPTION	EXAMPLES
PHYSICAL RISK	Anything that feels dangerous to your body	–Walking in a bad neighborhood –Turning off the lights –Touching a scorpion

TYPES OF RISKS

CATEGORY	DESCRIPTION	EXAMPLES
EMOTIONAL RISK	Experiencing, expressing, or exposing feelings	–Admitting fear –Proposing –Grieving a death
PROFESSIONAL RISK	Any gamble that pertains to your life's work	–Submitting a proposal –Writing a resume –Going back to school
SOCIAL RISK	Any situation where you are being judged by other people	–Performing publicly –Going on a blind date –learning a new skill in a group

If you don't know what risk you want to take, or if you're one of those people who claims to have no fears at all (yeah, right, and I'm Mahatma Gandhi), push yourself to take a risk in the category where you are *least* comfortable. Again, don't risk life, limb, or heartbreak just to say you did it; make sure your risk is necessary, take all possible precautions, and proceed very gradually.

Risk-Taking Step 2: Take the Smallest Scary Step Possible

One fine day, my client Paulette accompanied her husband, Henry, on a ski vacation. Paulette has an anxiety disorder and has never done well in situations that involve physical danger. Henry thought her uneasiness as a skier was just hilarious, so at one point, he tricked Paulette onto an expert-level slope, an absolute mess of cliffs, ice patches, near-vertical drops, and groves of trees. Paulette got back to the lodge an hour and a half later to tell Henry she was going to divorce him. And she did.

The point is that danger is best served in small portions. Research on phobias (not to mention common sense) shows that we lose our fears when exposed to so-called graduated risks. If you had a psychotic fear of bats, for example, a good psychologist wouldn't just ditch you in Carlsbad Caverns at dusk and hope for the best. Instead, you'd start by sitting down in a brightly lighted room and talking about bats for a while. With time, you'd become "de-conditioned to the stimulus"— in other words, the bat-chat would slowly become less a terror than an annoyance. Then the expert might show you drawings of bats until you felt comfortable looking at them. Then maybe you'd move on to viewing bat photographs, then maybe a dead bat, a bat in a cage, five bats in a zoo display, sixty bats in a convenience store, etc., etc. Given time, you'd be spelunking through hordes of flying mammals, maybe not with blithe indifference, but at least without paralyzing fear.

For Menu Item #5 to work best, you should break your risky action into tiny little doses. Most days, I complete this item just by writing a couple of paragraphs that are supposedly destined for publication, or worse yet, checking my e-mail, which always seems to contain a host of confusing demands. Today, as I've mentioned, is an exception; the smallest step that could really fulfill my heart's desire was a fairly large one. (I've now landed in San Francisco and checked into my hotel. I'll keep you posted as events transpire.) There will be days when you, too, will have to take a big jump instead of a tiny step. Just keep it as small as you possibly can.

**SOME GRADUATED RISKS (SMALLEST STEPS)
I COULD TAKE TOWARD MY HEART'S DESIRE**

_____

_____

_____

_____

_____

*Risk-Taking Step 3: Make Backing Out as Hard as
Going Forward*

The steps you've just listed are the kinds of moves you should
actually make. Do at least one of them today. If you agree with
me, but lack the motivation to get through your resistance, try a
nasty but effective little trick I like to play on myself and my
clients. It requires that while considering a goal from the security
of some literal or figurative armchair, you create structures that
will put your future self between a rock and a hard place, making
it as unpleasant to back away from a risk as it is to take it.

For many people, the most effective commitment structure
is peer pressure. For example, when I was an eighteen-year-old
college student, during a language drill in my Chinese class, I
tried to tell my fellow students that I was planning to run a
three-mile race. Unfortunately, my limited vocabulary and atrocious pronunciation wound up convincing my professor that I
was talking about the Boston Marathon. I had no idea how to
correct this misperception, so I just smiled and nodded as my

classmates made approving noises. Now I was stuck. During the ensuing months, when the weather was vile and my legs were tired and I didn't want to train, my mind's eye would conjure up the faces of my classmates and teachers, looking as disillusioned and disappointed as children Santa had failed to visit. Now, at an intellectual level, I knew that none of these people really cared whether or not I finished a marathon. Nevertheless, more times than I bothered to count, the thought of disappointing them goaded me into lacing up my shoes and heading out for a run. I actually did finish the big race that spring.

Committing to a group is probably the most powerful way to facilitate Menu Item #5. The more people who know about your promise, the better. However, remember that making a pact with a close friend is actually less motivating than declaring your intentions to relative strangers, as I did in Chinese class. That's because the more likely someone is to understand and forgive you, the more likely you'll be to weasel out of your commitment, confident that your loved one will give you a bye. I'm not saying this is psychologically healthy, I'm just saying that it works.

Another strong motivator is money. I used to do a lot of pro bono work, coaching unemployed clients for free, until I realized that these people never benefited much from my advice. Those who were paying good money were much more assiduous, because they wanted to make good on their investment.

You can become your own coach by spending money toward the risky steps you have identified. I once worked with a very talented writer, Mary, who had spent her adult life editing other people's work. She wanted to be a novelist, but her anxiety had stopped her from writing more than a few desultory paragraphs. During one session, I dragged Mary to a shop that sold nothing but expensive writing implements. Her assignment: to spend a ridiculous amount of money on a special pen, which she was to use only when writing her novel. Having forked over so much cash, Mary would feel as nervous and guilty about not writing as she did about facing the blank page. Even I was a little unnerved when Mary spent several hundred dollars (on a pen!), but I felt validated a few months later when the mailman delivered several gorgeously written pages of her first book.

My current version of Menu Item #5 was pretty much set in stone once I'd given my credit card number to the people at America West Airlines. Spending money meant that I climbed on the plane even though Isabella never answered the casual, how-ya-doin' message I left on her voice mail. Now it's midnight, and she hasn't called back—clearly, she prefers not to deal with me even as a disembodied voice. My mission of mercy has become a baneful intrusion. I plan to shoot myself as soon as my children are grown.

Risk-Taking Step 4: Don't Be Afraid to Be Afraid

As you can see, I tend to get a little hysterical in the midst of Menu Item #5, especially when the smallest risk that can move me forward is on the large side. I'll be fine, though, because fear doesn't scare me as much as it used to. I'm not joking. Fear does double damage if you're afraid to feel it: There's an initial reaction to whatever is scaring you, and then an additional resistance to feeling scared, which increases your anxiety level, which creates more resistance. . . . As anyone who's ever had a panic attack can attest, it can take just a few seconds for this self-reinforcing cycle to become incapacitating, full-on terror.

The way to ameliorate this problem, if not put an end to it, is to stop resisting your own fear. Accept the fact that you are going to be afraid at many times in your life, and decide that you'll be willing to experience this sensation, unpleasant though it is. When panic or anxiety arise, it helps very much to talk yourself through it. I mean literally. Do it out loud, if possible. Say things like "You're scared, and that's all right," or, "This is only fear, it won't kill me." I'm always surprised by how much this localizes the fearful sensations, as opposed to allowing them to generalize into an overwhelming terror.

Lao Tzu wrote, "Be like the forces of nature: when it blows, there is only wind; when it rains, there is only rain; when the clouds pass, the sun shines through." I thought about that in the autumn of 1987, when Hurricane Gloria made it all the way up the East Coast to my home in Massachusetts. That was an eerie day: The overcast sky turned a strange, bilious shade of yellow, and everyone who would ordinarily have been at work or school retreated behind boarded-up windows to wait out the storm. Early in the afternoon, the wind began to hum, then howl, then shriek. I watched it peel the aluminum siding off the house across the street as neatly as you'd peel an orange. And then it went away. Simple as that. That's what fear is like when you don't fight it. It's unpleasant as hell, but not nearly as unpleasant as the escalating feedback loop of resistance.

Risk-Taking Step 5: Walk into the Monster's Maw

One of the great heroes of Tibetan Buddhism, a man called Milarepa, once encountered a host of demons bent on driving him mad with fear. Some of them he chased away. Others he tamed with his huge compassion. But the biggest, meanest, ugliest monster of all simply would not leave until Milarepa, acting either on his profound intuition or a drug overdose, walked straight up to it and lay down in its mouth. As it swallowed him, the demon disappeared, and Milarepa achieved enlightenment.

Whenever you are contemplating a risk that is necessary to achieve your heart's desires, there will come a time when the only options are to live with a demon spirit—the ghost of a hope that will not leave you and will not die—or walk right into the thing that terrifies you most. After going through it a few times, you'll recognize such situations sooner, and walk toward the monster with less uncertainty. Oh, you'll still be scared. If you're doing something really important, you'll be scared beyond description. But you'll also feel the yearning to go on, fear or no fear. You'll find that you can follow that sweetness into the most dangerous undertakings, and that just as your terror destroys the person you used to be, someone stronger and braver always appears. It really doesn't matter what risk you take. The purpose of Menu Item #5 is to learn the strange, transformative magic of letting yourself be swallowed alive by whatever it is you fear.

Menu Item #5 Over Time

It has been several days since I traveled to San Francisco with delusions of Florence Nightingale dancing in my head. I went to bed that night at 2:00 A.M., having tried unsuccessfully to contact Isabella, embarrassed beyond words at having wasted my time and money offering support to someone who didn't want it. But just as I was turning out my hotel-room lights, my cell phone rang. It was Isabella, who had awoken in the middle of the night thinking, "Martha's in San Francisco." I headed for her apartment, just to be a warm body, someone to sit watch while she slept.

The results from Isabella's medical tests have just come back. They reveal that her alarming symptoms were caused not by cancer, but by an unusual bacterial infection. I hope my little odyssey helped my friend trust that she will never be alone in the world. Whatever its effect on her, though, my trip was a blessing for me. At this moment, I'm free from the regret I know I would feel if I'd simply spent that evening imagining what it must be like for Isabella to spend that night alone, facing the darkness, the memories of her mother's death, and an uncertain future.

So this version of Menu Item #5 turned out to have a happy ending, but that really isn't the point. The point is that, having followed my real desires instead of fear or social convention, I feel more whole, more myself, than if I'd backed away from the risk. For better or worse, every iteration of Menu Item #5 teaches you something useful: either that the world is safer than you thought, or that you can suffer disappointment and survive.

Oscar Wilde once wrote to a friend that "hearts are made to be broken." I've included that line in about twenty articles, and every time, my editors have cut it out. Apparently, it just doesn't sell magazines. But Wilde's point wasn't that we will always feel sad; it was that when we follow love rather than fear, we risk suffering the kind of heartbreak that allows us to grow, rather than crippling us. Pushing away our innate desires lacerates the heart so badly that it may not be able to recover; consciously risking heartbreak en route to the fulfillment of those desires actually makes us stronger. The heart is a muscle, and as any weight lifter knows, muscles grow stronger and more fit if they are torn just a little bit, then allowed to heal. Make no mistake: Putting your heart out into the world by taking risks for your true self means that it will be broken—and it will heal stronger than it was when you began. Refusing to risk is like allowing a muscle to atrophy; it doesn't hurt, but when the muscle isn't fulfilling its purpose, it loses whatever strength it has. The kind of heartbreak that comes from risking enough to claim your true desires is not the opposite of joy, but one of its components.

Further Adventures

If you practice Menu Item #5 every single day, the fear-walls that circumscribe your life will be pushed back, and back, and back, giving you more space in your life as a whole, as well as moving you toward fulfillment of your desires. You'll lose your fear of the little risks that once affected your choices, and things you once thought undoably huge will come to seem possible. Over time, you'll find that you have to extend your boundaries a long way to meet the requirements for Menu Item #5, because it will become harder and harder to find things that scare you.

For example, my client Steve decided to use this Joy Diet technique on his fear of heights, which, though not crippling, was intense enough to make him avoid standing on balconies or driving on mountain roads. He took a big risk by signing up for a climbing course at a local sporting-goods superstore. The first time he went up the climbing structure, Steve climbed about fifteen feet, then panicked, froze, and fell off. His belay line caught him and the instructor lowered him to the ground. Paradoxically, this experience gave Steve the beginnings of confidence in his equipment, and on the very next try, he got all the way up the wall. He did this every few weekends until he actually started to like it—no, make that love it. The little charge of adrenaline Steve got from the remnants of his fear made the experience downright exciting. To feel like he was really taking a risk, he eventually had to start climbing outdoor rocks, then really really big outdoor rocks, then honest-to-goodness mountains. Steve is still afraid of heights, but now we're talking about heights of a thousand feet or more, heights that would put any normal person into a fear-induced coma. Furthermore, he's so used to challenging his fears that when he sets out to master a difficult rock face, Steve just shrugs and moves right along, scared, careful, but undaunted.

Menu Item #5 will not eliminate fear from your life. Nothing can. But a daily risk can turn that fact from a torment into a blessing. It will expand your horizons, your confidence, your relationships, your achievements, and your happiness so much that in time, you will go looking for the shiver of apprehension that says you have reached the boundary of your comfort zone. You'll be pleased to reach the cusp between daring and fear, because you'll know from experience that that's where all the magic happens.

MENU ITEM #5: RISK

MINIMUM DAILY REQUIREMENTS

At least once a day:

1. Choose any scary goal. Name an action step you've devised for obtaining one of your heart's desires. Make sure that you really want this to happen, and that it really scares you.

2. Take the smallest scary step possible. Can your action step be broken down into smaller component parts? Determine the very smallest forward movement you can make.

3. Make backing out as hard as going forward. Commit your pride, your time, or your money to obtaining your ultimate goal. Announce your objective as publicly as possible.

4. Don't be afraid to be afraid. Accept that you'll be afraid as you take this step. Calm yourself with accepting and reinforcing self-talk.

5. Walk into the monster's maw. As Eleanor Roosevelt said, "You must do the thing you think you cannot do." Take a deep breath and jump.

TREATS

•

EVERY DAY, GIVE YOURSELF AT LEAST THREE REALLY GOOD TREATS: ONE FOR EVERY RISK YOU TAKE, AND TWO JUST BECAUSE YOU'RE YOU. NO EXCEPTIONS, NO EXCUSES.

YES, IT'S TRUE: YOU REALLY CAN TEACH A PIG TO push a shopping cart, and you don't even have to show him how.

I learned these glad tidings in a psychology textbook that featured an actual photograph of a cart-pushing pig, his fore-trotters poised delicately on the handlebar, a look of tremulous hope in his fine brown eyes. The hope was there because the pig was hungry, and the researchers who had locked him in a room with the shopping cart kept tossing him bits of food—but only when he did certain things. At first, they'd given him a treat every time he wandered near the cart. Then they began withholding the reward until he was actually touching the cart with some part of his body. After a while, the pig only received treats when his front feet were on the basket, then the handle-bars. In the end, just by reinforcing certain randomly occur-ring behaviors, the researchers had their porcine pal strutting around the room, pushing his cart as competently as any sea-soned Kmart shopper.

The researchers who conducted this experiment were from a psychological school known as behaviorism. They were test-ing the major hypothesis of their founder, B. F. Skinner, which is elegantly simple: Any animal will repeat behaviors that are positively reinforced (in other words, associated with some kind of reward or gratification), and avoid behaviors that are negatively reinforced (followed by pain, punishment, or dis-comfort). Though I personally think behaviorism is a bit too simplistic to fully explain the subtleties of human psychology, its basic premises are sound, and you're about to use them as part of the Joy Diet.

This chapter explains how you can literally train yourself to realize your best life by reinforcing yourself with a personal-ized repertoire of Menu Item #6: treats. I discuss how you can identify the treats that are most powerfully reinforcing to you, and how you can use them to profoundly alter your everyday behavior. Thus, by tossing yourself the pig chow of highly motivating rewards, you will learn to push the grocery cart of your life down the brightly lit aisle of destiny, undeterred by the wandering right wheel of self-destructive habits or the annoying clanking noise of misplaced socialization, all the while sampling freely from the nicely packaged consumer goods of joyful experience.

Why Treats Are Necessary

Most of the menu items on the Joy Diet are consistently pleasur-able in and of themselves. However, the menu item you've just completed, risk, can drain your psychological and physical energy and is often connected to danger, failure, disappointment, and fear—some of the most wildly negative stimuli you can imagine. Of course, the successes you'll encounter as you begin obtaining your heart's desires are so positive that they'll be enough to keep you going through enormous difficulty. Having just one dream come true makes almost any risk seem trivial, like the cost of a lottery ticket compared with the hundred-million-dollar jackpot. But big successes may not happen immediately, or often, and I don't believe in deferring gratification until that time. It's boring, and it simply doesn't work.

For instance, I've been taught for decades that restricting my diet to organic vegetables and exercising diligently would make me healthier, smarter, better-looking, and more beloved by the masses, but did that keep me from eating six large chocolate-chip cookies by nine o'clock this morning? It did not. My reasoning went like this: "Now, let me think. On one hand, there's my health. On the other hand, there are cookies. Health, cookies: cookies, health. Health . . . COOOOKIIIII-EEEES!" In short, I literally think like a pig: My behavior, while somewhat modified by long-term planning, is powerfully shaped by immediate rewards.

This is understandable when you consider that I am, after all, an animal. No offense, but so are you. Your body—including your brain—has a highly specific inborn agenda, and this includes pursuing short-term rewards even when they may not lead you toward your long-term objectives. Compared with other animals, humans are amazingly good at deferring gratification, but like every other creature tested by our friendly behaviorists, we eventually tire of doing things that bring no apparent gratification at all. If you've read my last book, you already know that I recommend bribing yourself to perform unpleasant but necessary tasks. The Joy Diet requires that you build on this strategy, waging an orchestrated campaign of reinforcement-based training. The idea is to lock in Joy Diet behaviors as habitual responses, so that you do them consistently without having to think much.

For example, my beagle, who, in accordance with our family obsession, goes by the name Cookie, gets a special snack every day at about four o'clock. In an unsuccessful attempt to keep our carpets clean, we always make Cookie eat this tidbit on an area rug that has a complicated pattern and therefore (theoretically) doesn't show spots. Cookie has no concept of carpet cleanliness, and for a long time he seemed confused about the fact that we wanted him to eat on the area rug. After a while, though, he became so used to having his treat there that now he feels uneasy eating it anywhere else, or straying far from the rug between suppertime and sundown. The other day, when we took the rug itself away to be cleaned, Cookie nearly fainted.

The risks, drudgery, and difficulty you must face to achieve your dreams are the "area rugs" (and by that I mean the "shopping carts") of your right life: They may feel strange or even repellent at first, but once you repeatedly associate them with something that's powerfully motivating to you, they'll come to seem comfortable, likable, even indispensable. Treats are the only way to create this training effect, and for that reason the Joy Diet requires that you reward yourself with a treat immediately after taking your daily risk. But treats also have another important function: They provide enough consistent short-term gratification to sustain the trust and happiness of the well-meaning animal that is your body. Giving yourself two treats a day whether or not you've done anything to deserve them is a crucial part of the Joy Diet. I'm so serious about this that I literally fire clients who won't commit to it.

Treating Yourself Right

I've mentioned that the treats you give yourself on the Joy Diet should be personalized. The assortment of rewards that motivate you most is unique to your physiology and personality; what seems like a treat to one person may actually be aversive to someone else. For example, you might be thrilled if someone offered you a trip to the gambling casinos of Las Vegas, while I would prefer being eaten by wolverines. So the first step toward completing Menu Item #6 is to develop a list of small delights—just little tiny ones—that reflect your particular preferences.

I'm astonished at how many people have trouble doing this. When I ask my clients to list their favorite treats, most of them look at me as though I've demanded that they tell me the Urdu word for "phlegm." Many can't come up with even one item. In general, the more high-achieving the client, the more slowly and patiently I have to explain the basic definition and identifying characteristics of these mysterious things I call treats. Since you're reading a self-help book, I'm going to assume that you're a member of the High Achievement Club, and begin at the beginning. Here, then, is the Joy Diet definition of the word *treat,* which may or may not correspond with your usual understanding of the word:

THE JOY DIET DEFINITION OF "TREAT"

Treat: Anything that makes you feel like smiling.

Some people seem surprised when I tell them this definition, mainly because of its emphasis on smiling. I began using it after reading the work of monk and activist Thich Nhat Hanh, who writes a great deal about smiling and claims, "If a child smiles, if an adult smiles, that is very important." Most of my clients don't believe this. After all, they argue, most humans smile hundreds of times a day, for a host of reasons (and we're not the only ones; Cookie is smiling at me right now, which I suspect means he is plotting insurrection). This is absolutely true. We get so used to pleasantly baring our teeth as a matter of social propriety or expediency that our smiles become as meaningless as a prostitute's caress.

But a socially appropriate, unfelt smile is very different from a spontaneous one. A genuine smile, like a sneeze or a yawn, instigates itself and is not totally under your control. It goes along with a certain inner sensation, different for each of us but unmistakable when you feel it. For you, it may be a sense of bubbling pleasure, or a tendency to hum, or a little tickle in your heart. You may not always smile when you feel it, but you certainly wouldn't mind. By contrast, any other sort of smile is a small violation of the true self.

Don't believe it? Try this: Put on a big old smile, right now. How does that feel? If you were in a pretty good mood already, it may have brightened you up even further, like an emotional tickle. If you're seriously unhappy, however, you'll probably find that smiling feels not only like an effort, but a betrayal. Call up the memory of a situation where you felt you had to smile even though you were sad or in pain, and you'll likely recall a sense of profound violation. Smiling is very serious business to our bodies and hearts, and to practice this part of the Joy Diet, you must treat it with respect. So . . .

Treat Step 1: Compile a List of Spontaneous Smile Sparkers

Start Menu Item #6 by simply observing your own smiling patterns for a day or two. Don't make any effort to control yourself; just watch. Can you feel what it's like when a smile bubbles up (whether or not you actually grin)? Are most of your smiles calculated to have some social effect, or do you find yourself beaming even when there's nothing to be gained by it? Is it different when you feel smilish because you find something funny, see someone you love, or succeed in some endeavor? Most important of all, when do you feel a spontaneous tendency to smile? Are your spontaneous smiles brief and fleeting, or do they ever seem to come all the way from your toes?

If you discover that you never feel like smiling at all, you don't just need the Joy Diet, you need serious help. I'm not kidding. Please go talk to a therapist, to see what situational or chemical imbalance is leaching the happiness out of your life. You may well be clinically depressed, and refusing to seek therapy or medical treatment for depression is about as brave and admirable as sticking yourself in the eye with a nut pick. Get help now.

If you aren't depressed, a few hours of observation should produce a list of events, situations, people, and objects that spark the sensation of an inner (and possibly an outer) smile. Write down all you can remember, on your own paper or in the following space. Go for at least ten—to start. If you can't come up with that many, vary your activities for a few days, remaining alert for smile sightings.

SMILE CATALYSTS

Some of the things that make me feel like smiling spontaneously are:

1. _____

2. _____

3. _____

4. _____

5. _____

6. _____

7. _____

8. _____

9. _____

10. _____

If you've been watching carefully and your list is still short,
you have probably been denying yourself treats far too long.
Many people who are just starting this phase of the Joy Diet
tend to come up with one or two Old Faithful items that sig-
nify luxury or indulgence to them. Frequently featured are the
standard treats you'll find in every women's magazine on the
planet: massage, hot baths, candles, pedicures. There's nothing
wrong with these things—I love them all, myself—but if
they're the only line items in your schedule that make you
smile, you haven't yet begun to reward the hopeful pig who
waits within you, hoping for a real, custom-made, individual-
ized treat. It's time to listen to your inner swine.

Treat Step 2: Indulge Your Beastly Self

In the poem "Wild Geese," Mary Oliver writes: "You only have to let the soft animal of your body love what it loves."

If you're like most civilized folk, this image may be quite arresting. You're probably not accustomed to thinking of your body as a "soft animal," much less one that should be allowed to love what it loves. My clients tend to push back against this idea, getting especially cerebral when told to reward their animal selves. "What would feel good?" I ask, and they reply, "I think it might be nice to see more foreign films," or, "I should probably try to work out more." These are thoughts, not feelings. They come from the nasty Nazi commandant of the superego, not the fleshy Bohemian beast that allows you to vividly experience both pleasure and pain. If seeing foreign films or working out feels so good to you that the very thought of doing so "smiles" you, then and only then are you allowed to put these things on your list of treats.

In the meantime, try greasing the wheels of your reward-detection machinery by going through your five senses, and naming things that delight each one. Have a go at this right now.

CATALOG OF SENSORY DELIGHTS

Finish each statement by listing five things that give you sensory pleasure.

1. I love the taste of: _____
_____
_____
_____
_____

2. I love the sight of: _____
_____
_____
_____
_____

3. I love the feel of: _____
_____
_____
_____
_____

4. I love the smell of: _____
_____
_____
_____
_____

5. I love the sound of: _____
_____
_____
_____
_____

You will probably find that your senses delight in rare and pricey things, like fine champagne or luxury vacations. But I've never had a client whose inner animal didn't also mention things that are simple and free: the light that slants through your shutters at sunset, the purr of a cat, the sensation of lying down and letting all your muscles relax at once. Your mind is likely to tell you that even these things—perhaps especially these things—are still too "expensive," that they require time and attention you just by God do not have. Examine these thoughts carefully. Notice the energy you feel when you think them. It's probably critical, judgmental, and tense (remember the signs of a false desire?). This is a sign that you are at war with your animal and probably have been for years. What you may not realize is that your animal is fighting back, and it usually wins. Take a few minutes three times a day to indulge it, and you will find that the primal forces of your mind and body begin to work for you in ways you've never experienced.

I've been telling people this kind of thing for years, but it still feels strange when it happens to me. For instance, one day I set out with my laptop, planning to hunker down in a coffee shop and write an article that wasn't coming together, no matter how hard I worked on it. About halfway to my destination, I found myself driving onto the wrong street, heading in the wrong direction. I felt strangely out of control, though I knew exactly where I was going: to the largest art supply store in Phoenix.

Understand that I take more sensory delight in the colors and textures of art supplies than almost anything on earth, but I hadn't even thought about buying any for years, since I became a busy working mom. I was fascinated and a little frightened by the intensity with which my animal body ended the art-supply drought. When I opened the door of the shop, the smell of paint, turpentine, cotton rag paper, charcoal, and rubber erasers literally stole my breath and brought tears to my eyes. I watched myself rush through the aisles tossing canvases, palette knives, and tubes of color into a (key phrase) shopping cart. The whole time, my mind kept repeating: "I don't have time for this, I don't have time for this, I don't have time for this." But it was wrong. After I left the store, with my wallet quite a bit lighter and my artsy fever somewhat abated, the article I'd been struggling to write popped out within an hour, like an egg—apparently, my inner animal is as much chicken as pig.

Ever since this experience, I've noticed that allowing myself to play with paint, to touch and see and smell this stuff I find so enchanting, brings my body and brain into a kind of alignment, making me much more productive in every other aspect of my life. I've found ways to work this into my schedule, carrying a small kit of art supplies in my purse, drawing or painting on airplanes, dabbling away while I'm on the phone. When I do this I'm more likely to accomplish my objectives, and life as a whole feels much, much more interesting.

I recommend that you put as many sensory pleasures into your schedule as you possibly can (three a day is an absolute minimum). In particular, interweave your least favorite activities with sense-pleasers. Buy a nine-dollar personal cassette player and listen to your favorite music while you do the dishes. Wear your favorite cologne whenever you pay the bills. If you have to meet with an unpleasant coworker, do it at your favorite restaurant, while eating your favorite dish (but watch it with this one, because if you rob it of other sensory pleasures, your animal self may use food as a panacea). Reexamine your list of sensory delights right now, and imagine ways you can include them as part of your daily life, particularly the parts of your daily life that feel boring or frightening.

I've watched dozens of clients improve their productivity and joie de vivre by using this technique. Indulging your senses is like being both the behaviorist research team and the pig with the shopping cart. You'll find that dreary or risky tasks become far more tolerable if you use your intellect to reinforce the useful behaviors of your animal self, rather than trying to logically persuade the animal to follow rules it doesn't know, acting on orders from people it can't understand, for a purpose it cannot imagine.

Treat Step 3: Practice Divine Decadence

This is far and away my favorite technique for identifying good treats. Begin by asking yourself what human virtues you most embody. Are you known for being patient, or competent, thorough, brave, trustworthy, clean, helpful, sensitive? Write down the qualities you think are your strengths, or those that other people find impressive:

MY SALIENT VIRTUES

Complete the following sentences:

1. People often compliment me on my ability to

_____

2. I am proud that I have the discipline to

_____

---

3. I am more virtuous than other people when it comes to

_____

4. Even when I don't feel like it, I always try to be

_____

Now, we're going to use your answers to practice divine decadence. This consists of doing something—or better yet, several things—that fly in the face of the virtues you embody. The reason for this is that, as the saying goes, "a strength exaggerated becomes a weakness." The stories we tell about ourselves are often based on an idealized image of perfect behavior that actually contradicts our real nature—otherwise, we wouldn't have to remain so conscious of it, or reinforce it with so much judgment. As I've worked with hundreds of clients, I've found that a person who talks on and on about being kind and gentle is probably repressing so much anger that he eventually becomes what I call an exploding doormat, holding back all assertiveness until he blows up in a real rage. A client who constantly refers to herself as "hardworking" will drive herself until she's physically ill. Someone who is obsessed with being a good Christian may get so self-righteous he attacks people in ways Christ never would.

The antidote to this form of excess is to mix a little dose of the libertine Mr. Hyde (he was the bad one) into your own virtuous Dr. Jekyll behavior. I once heard health guru Dr. Andrew Weil say that when he gets tired of being the perfect healthy eater, he likes to drink a Coke straight from the can. This is the kind of treat that can make virtue much more fun to sustain. If you're known for being tidy, start a project that will make a big mess (like throwing ceramics or building model airplanes), and spend a couple of days putting all your energy into creating before you even start to clean up. If you're incredibly responsible, call in sick for a noncrucial meeting and go to the movies. Doing this in areas where you are extraordinarily well-behaved will keep you from going off the deep end—I just want you to wade in the shallow end for a while. Here are a few examples of how you can balance virtue with delicious, harmless vice.

1. Be Unsophisticated

Patrick is one of the smartest people I've ever met. Like his father before him, he is literally a rocket scientist, as well as a brilliant writer with a gift for turning incomprehensible scientific ideas into pure poetry. Patrick's way of pursuing divine decadence is to put on a tank top and attend monster-truck rallies. He spends his time with the auto mechanics, asking the very stupidest questions he can think of. He tells me that this not only leaves him feeling fresh and energized but has led to several conceptual breakthroughs in his engineering work.

2. Be Profligate

I've read a lot of money-management books that mention how much of our hard-earned cash we could all save by, say, drinking instant coffee instead of blowing several dollars on specialty-shop versions. I suggest that if you're a really frugal person, you calculate these numbers carefully. Then go spend four bucks on a super-blended caramel malt-ball half-caff iced mochaccino. Give the counter guy a tip. If you want to get really decadent, let yourself actually enjoy it.

Obviously, you don't want to spend yourself into a financial crisis, but in my experience, small treat-splurges seem to go hand in hand with an increased ability to produce income. My favorite example is a client named Rosa, an incredibly frugal homemaker who, when I got to know her, couldn't buy herself a three-dollar bar of pretty soap (when she tried, she became overcome by anxiety and had to put it back). Rosa did eventually force herself to buy small treats. As she did, she suddenly began to see earning opportunities, from holding a garage sale to tutoring college students in Spanish, her native language. Within three years Rosa had made more income than she ever thought possible and was buying herself treats like expensive spa visits and a fancy touring bicycle.

3. BE IMMATURE

As a coach and mom, I spend a lot of time trying to be a reasonable, thoughtful, calm grown-up—except for the times when I am wildly, deliberately childish. I love finding bits of time in which I can spill, hide, play dress-up, and cry when I don't get what I want.

I also buy myself a lot of small, childish treats, like those gel pens with the sparkly ink. I was embarrassed at a recent book signing when I realized that I didn't have a single normal, black- or blue-ink pen with me. I asked the customers if I could borrow their pens, only to discover that about three-fourths of them were carrying their own pink and yellow and magenta gel pens. Indulge your childish side, and you may find that the world is full of immature, impulsive, playful, wonderful little kids, many of them disguised as adults.

4. BE IMMODEST

One of my former therapists (you'll be glad to know that I've visited several) used to start every session with "brags." Everyone in the office (it was group therapy, not schizophrenia) had to recount one story about something good they had recently achieved, completed, won, earned, or experienced. The more immodest the brag, better. Try to find at least one person with whom you can form a bragging compact. Get together with this person, and praise yourselves like professional athletes on a steroid high. Compare yourself favorably to your competition. Scorn all those who undervalue you. Be as conceited as you know how to be, until your brag session is over.

5. BE UNPRODUCTIVE

A friend of mine recently e-mailed me a very simple, very repetitive computer game, which is played by lining up rows of "jewels" in a large matrix. The thing about it is, the jewels are really shiny. Once I learned how the game worked, I spent so much time playing it that I developed tendonitis in my thumb. I called my friend, who is a high-powered businessman with a productivity level similar to Martha Stewart's, and complained that sending me a game with sparklies in it was like giving heroin to an addict. I told him, accusingly, about my thumb injury.

My friend laughed out loud, which I took to mean he was amazed that anyone could spend time as wastefully and unproductively as I had been doing. I was wrong; he laughed because he was nursing exactly the same injury, for exactly the same reason. Talking to him reminded me of something I should have remembered all along: that the occasional period of wasteful divine decadence is a treat that gratifies the true self and results in increased productivity over the long run.

This short list barely begins to cover the options for divine decadence. Go back to your list of virtues, and you can brainstorm dozens of ideas for becoming your own opposite for short periods, whenever you need a treat. You might enjoy

occasionally being insincere, lazy, slovenly, boring, cowardly . . .
go through a list of adjectives until you find one that brings a
spontaneous smile to your lips. Then, go for it.

Treat Step 4: Portion Out the Treats

Any good behaviorist will tell you that training an animal by
reinforcement requires careful portioning of treats. They must
come rarely enough to seem special, but frequently enough to
maintain hope. You can add as many small treats to your life as
possible, but for Menu Item #6, choose a few special ones that
aren't so easily accessible that they don't feel special. *Always give
yourself a treat as soon as possible after completing your daily risk.*
This will not only reward you for going after one particular
heart's desire, but also for daring to risk in general.

Aside from risk-rewards, I like my clients to give themselves one treat early in the day, and one in the late afternoon.
If you're busy, find ways to combine your treat with other
activity, the way I paint while I'm on the phone. Buy books-
on-tape (or check them out from the library) and listen to
them during your commute. Window-shop while you take a
walk that counts as your daily exercise. Call your best beloved
for a quick, gratifying exchange of unsophisticated baby-talk
while you're eating lunch. Whatever you do, find a way to
administer at least one treat in the morning, one in the afternoon. Remember, you can't train an animal with excuses or
evasion. Animals, including the animal part of you, only know
whether or not they are being rewarded. Honor your treat
agreements unless you are physically dead.

Treat Step 5: Outwit the Opposition

If you have a normal life, you're likely to encounter resistance when you set out to give yourself regular treats. The most serious opposition is likely to come from your own overactive conscience, from the part of you that is shocked and offended by self-indulgence.

To counteract this problem you need one simple thing: permission. The interesting thing is that you can get this from almost anyone. I know two successful and accomplished women, now both in their late sixties, who have mastered the art of self-reinforcement, but still occasionally need permission to treat themselves right. Whenever necessary, Meryl gets her permission from Barbara, and Barbara gets hers from Meryl. "We've been doing it for years," Barbara told me. "I'll call Meryl and say, 'I need permission to skip my grandson's piano recital.' She'll say, 'Barbara, why the hell would you want to go to a piano recital when you could be shopping?' It works like a charm every time."

If you have a great deal of resistance to giving yourself treats, find a Meryl or a Barbara. Get permission from your brother, your spouse, your friendly neighborhood life coach, this book—wherever you can find it. By the way, be very selective about whom you ask for permission. If you try to put your workaholic partner or your unforgiving mother in this role, you could end up mistreating yourself very badly. You should not only refrain from involving these people in your program of self-training, but keep the whole thing secret from them. The covert nature of the operation makes it even more fun.

The level of enjoyment my clients and I tend to get from three treats a day is often disproportionate to the small size and humble nature of the treats themselves. I've seen dozens of people go from lifeless-looking lumps to jolly, radiant adventurers just by sitting in my office and *promising* themselves treats. It works as long as they're willing to keep those promises, to keep tossing themselves the little bit of chow it takes to keep their animal selves excited and grateful.

What I love best about that famous cart-savvy pig is that no one had to model his unusual behavior for him; he just did whatever trick it took to get his treat. You may find that if you reinforce your own animal self by giving it a treat whenever it moves you closer to fulfilling your heart's desires, you'll end up doing things you never really expected. Maybe you've never seen anyone achieve that particular objective, create that particular effect. Maybe nobody ever has. Maybe you'll realize a destiny that is completely and uniquely yours, that will delight and surprise not only you but the rest of the world as well. And that, I promise you, is a major treat.

MENU ITEM #6: TREATS

MINIMUM DAILY REQUIREMENTS

Develop and deliver a set of personalized treats, using the following strategies:

1. Compile a list of spontaneous smile sparkers. Observe yourself for a few hours or days to see when you feel an "inner smile" (this may or may not result in a big old facial grin, but you'll feel that it could). Write down reminders of the things that make you smile spontaneously.

2. Indulge your beastly self. List several things that delight each of your senses. Go beyond the obvious or expensive to the small, subtle behaviors you may have overlooked.

Continued

3. Practice divine decadence. Consider the qualities about you that are most virtuous. Then, allow yourself to do something that is in complete contradiction to your virtuous self. If you are a neatnik, make a mess. If you're efficient, waste time. If you're conscientious, let something slide. You can go back to being virtuous when treat time is over.

4. Portion out the treats. You must always give yourself a treat as soon as possible after taking the daily risk specified in Menu Item #5. In addition, you should have one treat every morning, and one every afternoon or evening. If possible, weave more treats into your daily routine—but the first three are obligatory.

5. Outwit the opposition. If you find yourself resisting your treat regimen, bring someone else into the process. This person's job (as you'll explain) is to give you permission to treat yourself well, every single day. Keep the entire treat program secret from anyone you suspect may respond with criticism or judgment.

PLAY

•

**ONCE A DAY, TAKE A MOMENT TO REMEMBER YOUR REAL
LIFE'S WORK AND DIFFERENTIATE IT FROM THE GAMES
YOU PLAY IN ORDER TO ACHIEVE IT. THEN, COMMIT TO
PLAYING WHOLEHEARTEDLY.**

I HOPE YOU'RE ENJOYING TRAINING YOURSELF WITH
treats like the highly educable mammal you are. However, I'm
sure you're still aware that we humans are different from other
animals in key ways. For one thing, compared with most of our
planetary cohabitants, we're ridiculously inept. We don't have
the innate hunting ability of, say, a hawk or a tiger. Our defen-
sive skills are pathetic, too; we can't run very fast, we need a lot
of sleep, and we rarely smell predators creeping up on us, even
when they're wearing bad cologne. And yet humans have
become the dominant mammals on earth, because we have one
crucial quality all other species lack: We never grow up.

Anthropologists use the word *neotony* to describe the characteristics of very young mammals: relatively large heads, small
features, soft bodies, and, most of all, brains that are primed to
learn, learn, learn. Typically, the more intelligent the species,

the more pronounced the period of neotony is. For example, baby chimpanzees are extremely curious and quick. In fact, if you compare a human infant and a little chimpanzee born at the same time, the ape will learn and master new skills faster, at least for about a year. This is the age when a chimpanzee's brain switches from neotony to "adult" gear. Most of the chimpanzees you see wearing cute little suits on television haven't reached this stage, because once they go through it, chimps aren't nearly as attractive to the human viewing audience. They grow long, scary teeth. Their jaws and brows jut out. Their intelligence seems to "lock in," so that their learning curves slow drastically. They also become enormously strong, which makes it a tad frightening when their interests also shift, from learning adorable tricks to hitting people with trees.

Other primates, such as orangutans and gorillas, go through a similar transformation when they mature. But with the exception of my junior high school gym teacher, humans do not. Somewhere along the evolutionary road, we developed an aberrant mutation that makes us stay "babyish" all our lives. Even if we live a hundred years, we retain the general physical appearance of very young apes: small, rather delicate faces, large eyes, muscles much less powerful than those of our genetic cousins. Above all, we never lose the babyish qualities of inventiveness, curiosity, and the ability to problem-solve.

There's a word for the expression of these qualities. It's called "play." And if you know what's good for you, you'll do as much of it as you possibly can, forever. Menu Item #7 is designed to help you do just that. The remainder of this chapter explains why, when, and how.

When to Practice Menu Item #7

Be forewarned: If you stay on the Joy Diet for any length of time, you'll eventually reach a point where almost all of your time is spent playing. If this sounds good to you, you can start the process by simply creating a subtle shift in your perspective and attitude, a minimum of once a day. You'll do this by reviewing a few simple, self-evident facts that you know already, though, as with previous menu items, you may not be aware of them. This chapter walks you through the process that creates this shift in perspective. After that, you'll be able to do it again whenever you want—the more often, the better.

I suggest you create some sort of reminder to get you thinking about Menu Item #7 at least once a day. Monks in some Asian monasteries ring a bell at regular intervals, reminding everyone in earshot to stop, focus, and become wholly present for a moment. Even though their minds inevitably wander off again, the benefit of this brief, regular homecoming accrues steadily over weeks, and years, creating a pervasive inner climate of calm awareness. You can use any kind of "bell ringing" you like to remind you to practice Menu Item #7. Set an alarm clock or a beeping nine-dollar watch like mine, program a mnemonic phrase into your computer's screen saver, affix notes to your bathroom mirror, car dashboard, refrigerator, or significant other. Personally, I use surges of work-related anxiety as my trigger. Because it's so unpleasant, this kind of worry is highly motivating, and Menu Item #7 can help lessen it in just a few seconds.

Why and How to Practice Menu Item #7

Many of my clients stopped playing years ago. They wouldn't dream of doing anything they'd call "play," except on rare occasions like planned vacations or jury duty. They believe that play is inimical to success, that allowing themselves to play would cause them to lose their competitive edge at work. This is incredibly ironic when you consider that the play-intensive nature of our brains is the very thing that's allowed us to out-compete every other species on earth. A playful mind-set allows you to master whatever is in front of you, to form symbiotic alliances and partnerships, to adapt successfully to any challenging situation, and above all, to find a sense of fun that makes the whole shebang intrinsically satisfying. Play is precisely what you need most to succeed at work. It will also immeasurably improve your personal life, but as far as I'm concerned, the main reason to practice Menu Item #7 is that it's extremely, vitally, pivotally good for your career.

If you are unemployed and think you have no career, or if you have a job and assume I'm talking about that, think again. I'm using the word *career* to mean (as Webster puts it) "the course of action a person takes over a lifetime." When I say "your career," I'm referring to something you may never have worked on, even if you slave away at a job ninety hours a week: the course of action your true self would take if you were to live to the limit of your potential. I've had many clients who pursued impressive professions for years without ever coming near their real careers. Jerry went to medical school and became a radiologist, but in his heart, he's a Japanese scholar. Darlene is a dental hygienist, but she didn't feel complete career satisfaction until she married a widower and became mother to his two toddlers. Jessica is a retired air force captain who never did become a scientist, even though she always felt it was her real calling. Menu Item #7 starts with identifying your real career, even if you've never done anything related to it.

Play Step 1: Figure Out What Your Career Really Is

Recently, I figured out a shortcut to helping people conceptualize their real careers. I wish it weren't available, but since it is, we might as well use it. Just answer this question: What did you do on the evening of September 11, 2001? What seemed most important to you at the end of that terrible day?

I began asking clients this question after talking to several friends who were in Manhattan when the terrorist attacks occurred. That morning, all my friends were focused completely on things they considered very important. My friend Paul was trading stocks. Erica was editing the manuscript of a book. Larry was training for a bicycle race. My brilliant but troubled client Tracy was in a drug-induced fog, trying to cope with an ugly divorce. I've heard each of them describe what happened next: how they got The News, what they saw with their own eyes or on television, how they reacted. Their descriptions of the city that afternoon sound like science fiction: Hosts of silent New Yorkers all walking in the same direction, buying every pair of sneakers in town to substitute for high-heeled and dress shoes. Cars left with the keys in the ignition and the doors wide open, the radios blaring at top volume so that the migrating crowds could hear the latest news as they walked.

In the midst of this apocalyptic strangeness, each of my friends took some action that reflected his or her deepest values and true career. Paul, the driven financial genius, walked away from his window (which overlooked the Trade Center), turned off his computer for the first time since he'd bought it, and called his mother and girlfriend. Erica the editor began walking northward with the other people in her office, but not before she'd put the manuscript she'd been editing into her shoulder bag. Larry, who had been riding away from the Twin

Towers when they fell, turned his bicycle around and headed toward the smoking debris to see if he could help anyone who might be stranded or injured. Tracy drank a strong cup of coffee to clear her head, then went into the bathroom and flushed away several hundred dollars' worth of barbiturates.

My own reaction was to call my New York friends (all of whom were okay) and then to sit within touching distance of my immediate family members as we watched TV for several hours. My second impulse, which took over in the wee hours of September 12, was to begin fervidly composing magazine articles about the attacks, writing down what I'd learned from war survivors about how to cope with horror, outrage, and heartbreak. I was trying, in my lame way, to offer some kind of help to others—but I was also doing the things that felt most vital and real to me. In other words, connecting with my family, counseling, and writing are all parts of my true career. They were already my career (though I didn't know it) when I thought I would become a college professor—a fine job, but one that doesn't match my passions nearly as closely as the life I'm living now. There may come a time when my real career will take some new direction, and at that point, I'll have a choice: either to change my ways or lose a bit of myself. My real career has always been, and will always be, whatever action my heart and soul need to take. What I do for a living is just part of the structure I build to support this end.

So, what did you do on the evening of 9/11 (or during any time of severe crisis, the kind that divides your life into Before and After)? The answer is a very strong indicator of what your real career is, no matter what you do for money or how you spend your free time. Most career guidance counselors and time management schemes don't frame their questions starkly enough to get at the real issue in career selection. That question, as I see it, is "How do you want to live, given that you'll be dead pretty soon?" This kind of bluntness may appall you, but probably not as much as reaching the end of your life only to realize that you never really lived. Whether you live in New York or Brisbane or Antarctica, whether you're a soldier of fortune or an agoraphobe who hasn't left your apartment in twenty years, mortality will eventually claim you. When you think of that, what matters? What will you regret doing? What will you regret not doing? In the end, it boils down to two basic questions. You can answer them in the following box.

YOUR REAL CAREER

Please answer the following questions as honestly as you can.

1. When your life is over, how do you want the world to be different—in large ways or small—because you have lived?

_____

_____

_____

_____

_____

2. What experiences must you have to feel you've lived a completely satisfying life?

_____

_____

_____

Continued

_____

_____

THE ACTIVITES THAT WOULD ALLOW YOU TO ACHIEVE AND
EXPERIENCE THE THINGS YOU HAVE JUST IDENTIFIED—AND
ONLY THESE ACTIVITIES—COMPRISE YOUR REAL CAREER.

If you can find ways to create in reality the things you just
jotted down on paper, you will have had a brilliantly successful
career, even if you never make a dime. If you don't come anywhere close to realizing these goals, you will have failed at your
true career no matter how much wealth, power, and prestige
you manage to obtain. The first step in adding Menu Item #7
to your daily life is to remember what your real career is, to
consciously bring into your mind a vivid picture of the things
that would matter most to you if you knew you were going to
die. Because (big smile) you are! Have a nice day!

Play Step 2: Realize That Almost Every Sphere of Human Society Can Be Seen as a Game

Bringing up death to preface a discussion of playfulness really
isn't as incongruous as it may seem, because it is in the clear
light of honesty about our mortal condition that almost every
activity we humans conduct appears in its true form—as a
game. A game is an artificial situation including a stated goal
and a set of rules players must keep to reach that goal. That
describes almost everyone's job, and most nonprofessional pastimes as well. Unfortunately, we have a tendency to get so
involved in these games that we mistake them for reality. In the

instant that we do this, our lives become humorless and desperate, losing all the playfulness our true selves want to bring to our real careers. We feel as though we're struggling with a grim, unalterable reality, when we could simply be enjoying whatever game we've chosen with a relaxed awareness of its arbitrariness and ultimate unimportance.

Consider the way the events of 9/11 brought this into focus for my New York friends. Paul, the financial whiz kid, had always considered the stock market the realest part of real life. "I used to be so obsessed," he recalls. "I thought nothing else mattered." But in the aftermath of disaster—surprise, surprise—Paul found that his relationships were his real life, and stock trading was simply a game he liked to play. "I've been much more balanced since," he says. "The market has taken a horrific beating, but it just doesn't bother me like it would have before. My life is about my family."

A few blocks away from Paul's building, Erica the editor walked out of her office as well; the disaster made corporate busywork look about as crucial as a game of tiddledywinks. But Erica took the manuscript she was working on, because its content still mattered to her, and working on it was part of her real life, her real career. Doing it in a corporate setting was just a way she had found to play an interesting game that served her life's purpose. Larry, who had always lived to win bicycle races, found that this game meant very little to him, except insofar as it had given him strength and fitness with which to help people who were weak and injured. The role of helper was his real career. And Tracy, the spurned spouse, learned that even the interpersonal sparring between her and her ex-husband felt like a game, as did her use of drugs to manipulate her own emotions. What really mattered to her, it turned out, was being fully conscious and present, even in a condition of great emotional pain.

I'm not saying that the games these people were originally playing—business, competition, relationships—aren't significant or necessary. I work flat out every day to help my clients win such games, and to win them myself. But the first step to victory, and the only step that can make these games *fun,* is to see them for the essentially expendable conventions they are. You may have heard the wise saying that in any competitive situation, whoever has the least interest has the most power. When we know we're playing a game, we're less attached to the outcome, and therefore more powerful, than people who think their very souls are at stake.

I had my own little September 11 when I was in my twenties, deeply involved in a game called "academia." Being born and raised a faculty brat, and having spent my whole adult life as a Harvard student, I actually thought this game was my life. Then I had to make a choice about whether to bear a child who had been diagnosed, in my sixth month of pregnancy, with Down syndrome. Academia, fine old game though it is, suddenly seemed vanishingly insignificant. What mattered to me in the final analysis was the opportunity to love and learn with my heart, not my head. It was like breaking a spell: No matter how vociferously my advisers urged me not to throw away my future by keeping the baby, I could never again see the university system as my real career.

The strange thing was that I became much better at the game of academia after having this epiphany—even with my special-needs baby in tow. I made different choices, opting for projects that interested me even if they were low profile, hanging out with people I enjoyed rather than those who were best known in their fields. In short, I began playing only the parts of the academia game that felt fun to me, and ignoring all the things people told me I was supposed to do to get ahead. And yet, these choices always seemed to end up benefiting me more than anyone—including I—expected. The humble projects received surprise funding. The work I did with good friends was amazingly well received. The power of play was beginning to show up in my work.

Ever since, I have observed that in every professional discipline, there seem to be two types of extraordinarily successful people. On one hand, there are those who absolutely believe that the game they're playing is Real Life, who would kill or die to win. These people may dominate their games for a time by sheer force of will, but they often seem stressed and joyless, unable to feel satisfied even by their amazing achievements. On the other hand, there are the people who see very clearly that their profession is a game, but who simply love playing it. These people enjoy their successes with wholehearted delight and joke about their failures with sheepish good humor. They care about their work, but it is not the foundation of their happiness. They seem to dwell in what Roshi Shunryu Suzuki called "big mind."

> *To exist in big mind is an act of faith, which is different from the usual faith of believing in a particular idea or being. It is to believe that something is supporting us and supporting all our activities including thinking mind and emotional feelings. . . . That is the feeling of pure being.*

Call it whatever you want—God, truth, the consciousness of mortality, your real self—this ground of pure being is where you can stand to find peace when you are in danger of mistaking this or that game for your real life. Remind yourself of your true priorities at least once a day, when your Menu Item #7 reminder prompts you, and you'll gradually learn to return to this stable foothold more quickly and more often. Once you feel grounded, you can move on to the next stage of this menu item: testing to see whether the games you're playing are serving your real life.

Play Step 3: See Whether the Game You're Playing Is Useful for You

Many of my clients become very stressed about choosing the "right" profession, the "right" way to handle a relationship, the "right" company. They seem to believe that all the choices they make are hugely momentous, that there is only one perfect choice in any given situation. From the perspective of the true self, this is like thinking it's direly important whether you play Old Maid or Parcheesi for the next half hour. I've had many clients in the latter years of middle age who've never joined in anything wholeheartedly—not relationships, not professions, not even hobbies—because they're so afraid of making the "wrong" decision. Moving into the perspective of big mind will help you see through the illusion that every choice you make is earth-shatteringly important. Then you can walk away from unsuitable games without agonizing and join new ones without being paralyzed by perfectionism.

A number of criteria can indicate whether the game you're playing is working for you. Whenever your Menu Item #7 prompter nudges you back to attention, back to big mind, you might ask yourself the following questions.

DOES THE GAME YOU'RE PLAYING SERVE YOUR REAL LIFE?

- **Does playing this game contribute to my real career, or detract from it?**

If your real career is to be a healer and you get a chance to play the Registered Nurse game, or the Religious Leader game, go for it. Or you may decide to join a game (like, say, Bartending or Newspaper Delivery) that supports your purpose indirectly. However, do not join a game that will take you away from your life's purpose, *no matter what prizes are being offered*. If you spend your whole life playing a game that is not your real career, you'll lose even if you win.

• Am I having fun?

All Joy Dieters should take fun very, very seriously. Playing a game that supports your real purpose is fun the way a difficult sport can be fun; you may spill gallons of blood, sweat, and tears on the playing field, but you wouldn't trade the chance to do it for anything in the world. A game that's fun for you is worth playing, even if it's a huge effort. A game that isn't any fun at all had better serve your purpose fairly directly. If it doesn't, take the very next time out to start looking for a game that would suit your purpose better.

• Am I good at this game (or could I be good at it if I practiced)?

It's tempting to stay buttoned into things you do well, but if desire tells you to jump into a game you've never really learned to play, listen to it. The worst that can happen is that you'll lose. That's all right. It doesn't really matter, and we usually learn a great deal more from losing games than from winning them. If we just keep playing around, we almost always end up in a game that matches our innate abilities.

Continued

• **Do I like the other players? My teammates? My competitors? My coaches?**

Trust this: Whatever your life's purpose, hanging with people you love is part of it. Often, it's worth putting up with a grueling, often thankless game (such as Parenthood) in exchange for the chance to associate with extraordinary people (such as your children). People who share your passions, your talents, and your ambitions are more likely to be concentrated in games that will serve your real career. Playing games with them is almost always worth your while.

If the answer to *any* of the preceding questions is yes, go ahead and play your game wholeheartedly, without reservation, until you can make an even more informed judgment about its staying power. If you answer no on *every single point,* you're in a game that is actually detracting from your real purpose in life. This isn't a catastrophe—for heaven's sake, it's just a game!—but it should prompt you to start scouting the horizon for new games to play. If you stay curious and open, you'll find a more useful game soon enough. When you do, you'll have a lot more fun.

Play Step 4: Learn to Alternate Mouse Vision and Eagle Vision

In Sioux Indian culture, the eagle symbolizes the ability to see distant goals and vast scenarios with great acuity. The mouse is a metaphor for the state of mind that focuses completely on the thing right in front of it, putting all its attention on exploring whatever it is with eyes, nose, whiskers, and tiny little paws. The ability to move back and forth between eagle vision and mouse vision is the heart and soul of Menu Item #7.

When your alarm clock or screen saver or anxiety remind you that it's time for this attitude adjustment, stop and take a long look at whatever you happen to be doing: chatting with a colleague, putting gas in your car, composing music, whatever. Next, switch your focus to the major life goals you listed earlier in this chapter (the ways you want to change the world, and the experiences you need to feel your life is complete). Now, focus on the immediate task again. Switch back and forth a few times: real career, current task, real career, current task, eagle, mouse, eagle, mouse, eagle, mouse. Do the two things line up along the same trajectory? Is the smallest action you are taking moving you toward any of your ultimate objectives? If so, how efficient is it? In other words, does this action divert some of your energy into things that aren't part of your true career, or is it purely "on purpose" for you?

Some actions will lead straight toward your dreams (working out will help you finish that triathlon, paying attention to your partner will help you maintain a solid relationship, and so on). Other activities, like doing your taxes, cleaning your living room, or getting a flu shot, are basically maintenance work, meant to support more goal-directed efforts. That's fine, as long as you're not using mousy maintenance behaviors to substitute for your real career. When I hear a client say something like "I've been meaning to travel for years, but someone has to cook for my family," or "My job is killing me, but I have to pay the rent," I smell an overly influential mouse. Playing the martyr by doing maintenance work that keeps you eternally away from your eagle goals may be your way of dodging the scary, exhilarating work of your real career. Almost any maintenance problem can be circumnavigated with a little creativity. Let your family eat take-out for a week while you live your travel dreams. Find a new job—there are plenty of ways to pay the rent that won't snuff the life out of you. Keep thinking creatively and risking boldly until none of your mouse activities actually detracts from your eagle goals.

Performing the eagle vision /mouse vision switcheroo is like analyzing your golf swing or skiing turn to see how even your smallest actions may be contributing to or detracting from your overall performance. It's very important to be grounded in awareness of The Big Picture, but we can't achieve such grand goals except through a series of actions that may be broken down into tiny fragments, and each of these fragments is best accomplished if we give it full attention. Allowing yourself to focus completely on the smallest step is what ensures that you will eventually achieve even your most lofty goals. Reminding yourself to keep adjusting your behavior in light of the distant scene is what helps you play your games skillfully, assuring that they take you toward your ultimate purpose with a minimum of waste and effort.

If you notice that your present activity is contributing nothing to your larger objectives—in other words, if your mouse self isn't headed in the same direction as your eagle self—you must change course, but not by a huge degree. At the mouse-view level, you might readjust your behavior by spending five minutes on a task you were ignoring, or sending a single quick e-mail that leads toward your eagle-vision objectives.

For example, my client Monica is completely occupied with her six-month-old twins, but ultimately, she'd love to be in a job that involves a lot of travel. Her mouse-level adjustment for one day might be, say, going online to figure out how to get passports for the kids, so that when they're five or six and Monica starts playing the Business Traveler game, they'll be able to accompany her on some of her trips. Harold is in middle management for a major national bank, but he knows he's going to become a psychotherapist within the next few years. Observing the dynamics of the social interactions at the office and reading *Psychology Today* on the subway are two mouse-view activities he uses to brings his daily activities into line with his purpose. Very small adjustments like these add up to huge differences in trajectory as we play our various life games for months and years. In every game, the players who tend to win are those who move fluidly between eagle and mouse vision.

MOUSE VISION / EAGLE VISION

1. Summarize the real objectives of your life, as just discussed. Think *huge*.

_____

_____

_____

_____

_____

2. Now write down three small, mousey things you might do today to move closer to any of your objectives. Think *tiny*.

a. _____

b. _____

c. _____

Play Step 5: Be Like Water Flowing

When my son Adam was five years old, I took him to a karate class, hoping that he could learn to beat up anyone who might make fun of him because of his disability. When we got to the class, Adam showed no interest whatsoever in the martial arts. This reminded me of one of those truths I'd known all along, without realizing it: Adam is a completely nonviolent person. *I* was the one who wanted to beat up anyone who made fun of him. So I took Adam home and returned to karate class myself.

In the years that followed, I would become legendary in my local *dojo* for my distinctive wild flailing style and near-total inability to relax. "Loosen up, Dr. Beck!" my teacher would shout, respectfully using my title as I thrashed away, trying to sock some poor teenage boy who'd been forced to spar with me. "It's like a dance, Dr. Beck! It should be fun!"

I found this advice manifestly insane. For one thing, we were learning techniques like how to gouge out an attacker's eyes *en route* to ripping his facial bones off the rest of his skull—not part of the Hokey Pokey, last I checked. For another thing, I was smaller, older, and weaker than anyone I had to fight, so I felt I should compensate with extra effort. One day I explained this to my teacher, who rolled his eyes. "That's exactly why you have to be even *more* relaxed," he said. "It has to feel like playing your favorite game. If size and strength are against you, the only way to win is to be like water flowing."

This sounded pretty, but I still didn't believe it. Then one morning I was practicing some punches on the 270-pound, ground-standing heavy bag, and I got distracted by something I'd seen through the window. I threw out a last punch, a sort of half-hearted good-bye tap, and was shocked when the bag moved back about a foot. My hardest punches had barely jostled it, but what felt like a flick of my wrist had apparently taught it some respect. I was so excited I hauled off and pounded the bag as hard as I could. I almost broke my arm. The bag didn't budge. But in that one accidental moment, when I'd stopped fighting and started playing, I'd finally experienced how it felt to move like water flowing. From then on, I began focusing on what felt fun, rather than what felt strong. It's not like I became a world-class martial artist, but in all modesty I must admit that my hulking teenage classmates stopped calling me Dr. Beck and started calling me Mrs. Pain.

"When two great forces collide," says Lao Tzu, "the victory will go to the one that knows how to yield." This doesn't mean that we should give in to the opponents who face off against us as we play the various games of human existence. It means that we should surrender to relaxation, to flexibility, to the balanced state of mind and body that makes doing a job, raising a child, negotiating a deal, even violent conflict, feel like dancing. With this kind of surrender as our modus operandi, the exigencies of our jobs and responsibilities become like obstacles in the path of flowing water. We end up going over, under, around, and through all of them, always eventually finding a course that leads to our real lives, the way water always follows the pull of gravity. Fighting to make things happen the way we want them to prevents this response. Playfulness makes it possible.

Flow is the very word psychologist Mihalyi Csikszentmihayli used to describe the state in which people experience maximum enjoyment and maximum achievement. He found that our deepest pleasure doesn't come from total lethargy and ease. It comes from experiences that both interest and challenge us. Our always-childlike brains thrive on learning, puzzling, striving, and solving problems. Picasso said, "I have worked all my life to learn how to paint like a child." Menu Item #7 shifts your focus from dreading and avoiding difficulty to finding the sort of difficulty you can love, and making sure you don't take it too seriously. Do it consistently, and you will reach the point where there is no difference between your work and your play. And once that happens, take it from me, life is freakin' *fun*.

As you become more connected to your ideal blend of playful activities, you'll do Menu Item #7 more and more often, until you no longer have to make this mental shift— you'll live in the perspective of playfulness automatically. You can drop your prompters, your versions of the temple bell that rings to remind you—re-mind you—to stand on the ground of your deepest being. In fact, the whole world will remind you, because of the vibrancy and delight you'll find in playing, things you may not have experienced since childhood. As one poet put it in the sparse syllables of my favorite haiku:

> *The temple bell stops*
> *But the sound keeps on coming*
> *Out of the flowers.*

MENU ITEM #7: PLAY

MINIMUM DAILY REQUIREMENTS

Get a prompter of some sort to remind you to apply this menu item at least once a day.

1. Figure out what your career really is. Ask yourself what mattered to you most after you experienced or witnessed a genuine tragedy. Remind yourself that your real career consists of the changes you wish to make in the world and the experiences you want to have before your life is over.

2. Realize that almost every sphere of human society can be seen as a game. Notice that your job and many of your other activities are arbitrary systems in which people agree to follow certain rules to compete with each other, in order to win prizes like titles, money, and power. See that there are many possible alternatives to playing the game you happen to be involved in right now.

3. See whether the game you're playing is useful for you.

4. Learn to alternate mouse vision and eagle vision. When your Menu Item #7 prompter reminds you, stop and focus on the biggest, most important goals in your real life. Then, switch your focus to the task in front of you. Do they align? If not, you may need to adjust your immediate behavior slightly to create large changes in trajectory over time.

5. Be like water flowing. Once you are focused on your real objectives and have learned to see your progress toward them as a series of games, you will become more relaxed and playful, developing the flexibility and adaptability that makes children so resilient and quick to learn. You'll do whatever you try more effectively and successfully, and more to the point, you'll end up having more fun than you ever imagined.

LAUGHTER

•

**EVERY DAY, MAKE SURE THAT YOU LAUGH AT LEAST
THIRTY TIMES. IF THIS IS NOT POSSIBLE, USE THE
LAUGHTER ALTERNATIVES DESCRIBED IN THIS CHAPTER.**

HERE'S HOW MY OXFORD DICTIONARY DEFINES IT:
"The spasmodic utterance, facial distortion, shaking of the
sides, etc., which form the instinctive impression of mirth." To
me this sounds like the array of symptoms caused by a lethal
virus, but it's actually a description of one of the best things
life has to offer: laughter. With certain exceptions, the Joy Diet
requires you to do it at least thirty times a day.

If that sounds like a lot, consider that a typical small child
laughs over four hundred times a day. For the average adult, the
number is a paltry fifteen—but of course, you are not an average
adult. You are a Joy Dieter, with the dedication and discipline to
become way sillier than an ordinary person. After you've read
this chapter, I think you'll agree that doubling the average person's quota of laughs per day is the least you can ask of yourself.

If I'm wrong, and you're not up to the challenge of Menu
Item #8, I doubt you'll be able to stay on the rest of the Joy

Diet. This is because continually pushing yourself to become more authentic and adventurous, as the Diet requires, will take you to the edge of your comfort zone in a thousand different ways. Sometimes, especially when you're about to achieve some kind of breakthrough, you'll get stuck, paralyzed by anxiety or uncertainty. I believe that laughter is a kind of psychological Drano designed specifically for these situations. It breaks up mental clogs, allowing your thoughts, feelings, intuitions, and actions to flow freely into areas you may never have explored. The more you encourage yourself to laugh, the broader the horizons of your life will become. So let's take a very serious look at laughter, considering why, when, and how you can maximize your LPD (laughs per day).

Why Laugh? The Scientific Basis

There's an impressive amount of scientific research on the topic of laughter. First of all, you'll be glad to know that it has been studied and found safe in laboratory animals. I didn't even know that nonhuman creatures were capable of laughter, but it turns out they are. One study reported that rats and mice were willing to learn new tricks if they knew that when they were finished, scientists would reward them by reaching into their cages, rolling them on their backs, and tickling them. During this procedure, the animals made a noise that researchers identified as giggling, although, according to one report, "the sound is so different from us that it's hard to directly equate it with human laughter." The study does not mention whether anyone involved in this experiment, either human or rodent, had been doing a lot of recreational drugs. That is not important. What matters is that, having determined that laughter was gratifying for rats and mice, researchers went on to study it in nonhuman primates.

Apparently, our nearest genetic relatives are having a wacky old time out in the African bush, because they, too, enjoy a good chuckle. "Tickle a chimp or gorilla," says one study, "and rather than 'ha-ha-ha-ing,' they will gasp repeatedly. That's the sound of an ape having a good time." This begs the question of how the researchers *know* the apes are having a good time. If a bunch of scientists suddenly started tickling the pope, I imagine he'd gasp repeatedly, too, but not necessarily because he liked it. At any rate, these groundbreaking studies appear to have established that *homo sapiens* is not the only species with a strange predilection for spasmodic utterances. All manner of beings love to laugh.

You can see why this trait evolved when you survey the medical research on the way laughing affects the body. Laughter—even the anticipation of laughter—shifts our internal chemistry measurably, reducing stress hormones and increasing the number of natural virus-killer cells available to fight diseases from colds to cancer. It also triggers the release of endorphins, hormones that lessen the perception of distress and make us feel fabulous. The cliché is true; laughter really is very good medicine—so much so that some hospitals have "Laugh Mobiles," that hand out videotaped comedy routines and squirt guns to their patients. At a hospital in Oklahoma City, nurses are encouraged to use squirt guns on each other. Head nurses (this is true) get to use a Super Soaker. One assumes they restrain themselves while participating in procedures like brain surgery, but one would be intrigued if this turned out to be a false assumption, as long as one was not the patient undergoing the operation.

As powerful as the physiological benefits of laughter may be, however, it appears they are less important than the role laughter plays in social interaction. Laughter is like social glue; it binds people together and fills the small gaps that inevitably remain between them. Researchers who should know tell us that we laugh most often not because something strikes us as funny, but because we're trying to smooth interpersonal communication. One group of psychologists skulked around in malls for ten full years, ostensibly shopping for hair accessories, but actually writing down everything they heard people say just before "naturally occurring laughter." They discovered that laughter "usually was in response to statements like, 'Hey, how have you been?' or 'Do you have a rubber band?'" These are not exactly gut-splitting witticisms, but laughing at them softens communication, making conversation friendlier.

Living your right life is a process that needs the smoothing and bonding effects of laughter. Following a path that is uniquely yours means, by definition, that you'll sometimes go off in directions other people—including your friends and family members—will not fully understand. Being able to laugh with the people you love will make it possible for you to take unorthodox actions with minimal disruption to your relationships.

Without the physical and social effects of laughter, I, for one, would almost certainly be dead. I have spent a lot of time in the strung-out zone where death and laughter appear to be the only viable options. Without option number two, I'm pretty sure I would have succumbed to stress-related illness, checked myself out of the Terra Firma Hotel, or been gunned down by any number of people who have good reason to want me dead (the night manager at the All-Nite Chuckomatic, all lovers of fine writing, the woman who was PTA president at my children's elementary school during that regrettable incident with the cupcakes, etc.).

When Should We Laugh?

There's a counterintuitive fact that you must understand to implement Menu Item #8: *The more stressful, dangerous, baffling, or unpleasant your situation, the more important it is to laugh at it.* Fortunately, the very nature of humor lends itself to this strategy. The "tickle effect," the amount of hilarity produced by any given situation, seems directly related to how uncomfortable it makes us.

For instance, babies are innately afraid of being abandoned, especially since they lack the concept of object permanence—the understanding that when something disappears from their immediate perception, it still exists. One-year-olds laugh at peekaboo because it plays on their worst insecurities. An adult disappears, and baby starts to panic; then, boom! the adult is back again. The cutting edge of anxiety, followed by sudden reassurance, provokes gales of laughter. As we grow up, most of us eventually twig to the object-permanence thing, and peekaboo loses its hilarity. But we continue to laugh most at things that elicit anxiety. We find it funny when someone slips on a banana peel because falling down in public is an embarrassing eventuality we all hope to avoid. Comedians pad their routines and wallets with subjects like dating, family dysfunction, sex, and other topics about which most of us feel at least a little nervous. Any issue that pushes us right up to the boundary of our comfort zone is potentially amusing.

Of course, certain things are so painful that nothing about them is funny. However, these things are surprisingly rare. Several weeks after the destruction of the World Trade Center, humorists, TV personalities, and ordinary people began to make cautious jokes about the tragedy. Ellen DeGeneres got huge laughs when she explained why she was perfect for the job of hosting the disaster-delayed Emmy Awards. "What could bug the Taliban more," she told her audience, "than seeing a gay woman in a suit surrounded by Jews?" This one sentence alluded to a good half-dozen of the most distressing issues in American culture: terrorism, homophobia, religious fundamentalism, sexism, anti-Semitism, and fashion faux pas. You'd think we would want to avoid all these fraught topics during a celebration, but the opposite is true. Millions of people laughed at that joke, because making fun of such deeply upsetting problems was not only witty, but heartening. It showed that, as a people, we were stretching the boundaries of our cultural comfort zone enough to incorporate the fear and grief created by hate crimes of unprecedented awfulness. Laughing at the world post 9/11 was a sign that we were ready to handle it.

Speaking of Ellen DeGeneres, you may know that her biggest career breakthrough came in the wake of personal disaster, after her life partner was killed in a traffic accident. Twenty-three-year-old DeGeneres was grieving in a cheap hotel room when she wrote down a "conversation with God" that won a nationwide humor competition and landed her on the *Tonight Show*. On a far more modest scale, I also know how it feels to achieve success by chortling at tragedy. I once wrote a memoir that was (I hope) a chuckle-filled romp through a life-threatening pregnancy that ended with the birth of a mentally retarded baby. That experience was so wretched that even when it was happening to me—during a time when nothing could make me smile, much less laugh—I knew it could be hilarious in hindsight. The book sold surprisingly well, which convinced me that people will pay good money to be able to laugh at unpleasant circumstances. I encourage all Joy Dieters to join me in milking this quirk of human psychology for every red cent we can get.

Humor Fitness: Increasing Your LPD Quotient

I arrived at the thirty-laughs-per-day requirement only after my editor and I, in the bold if foolhardy tradition of committed scientists, experimented on ourselves. Since both of us are trained in research methodology, we did it right, carrying around two official-looking metal tally counters and clicking them every single time we laughed, except when we forgot. We forgot kind of a lot. Even so, our total was way over thirty laughs a day—we topped that number in the first half hour. True, these results were biased by our consumption of several scientific margaritas, my editor's appalling lack of reverence for the research process, and the fact that, as my thirteen-year-old daughter explained to an alarmed friend, "My mother is easily amused." Also, we were unaccountably amused by the act of clicking our tally counters—in fact, by the very phrase "tally counter"—so every time we clicked, we laughed, which meant we had to click again, which meant . . . you get the picture. Still, it convinced me that laughing thirty times requires no special effort or deviation from an ordinary daily routine. You can blend it in with practically any other activity.

A few major factors will determine how easy it will be for you, personally, to meet the Joy Diet laughter requirement. Some of the variation in individual laughter rates seems to be hereditary (consider the famous case study of identical twins raised apart, who were known to scientists as The Giggle Sisters because they both laughed almost continuously). Obviously, circumstances also contribute to determining individual LPD—you may laugh very little at the doctor's office, a lot when you're at your local comedy club or opium den. A third, more controllable factor is something I call humor fitness. Being humor-fit means that you deliberately and consistently find reasons to laugh, no matter what circumstances nature and nurture may hand you. People who are very fit laugh most at the one thing they'll always have around: themselves. The Joy Diet strongly encourages you to take command of your LPD rate by evaluating your natural laughter propensities, seeking laugh-enhancing circumstances, finding humor in situations where it may not be obvious, and learning to laugh at yourself. But before we discuss strategies for achieving this, it's time for a very important caveat.

Caveat: Emergency Laughter Alternatives

There are certain circumstances under which laughing is next to impossible. If you're suffering so intensely that you can't laugh, the Joy Diet requires that you substitute alternate forms of spasmodic-uttering, facial-distorting, side-shaking emotional expression: yelling or crying. Choose the first of these if you are filled with anger, the second if you're overwhelmed by sorrow, and either one (or both) if the problem is fear. This requires a bit more time investment than the standard Menu Item #8, but if you're too upset to laugh, you desperately need to do it.

You can conduct your laughter alternative in the company of an understanding loved one, or all by yourself. Just go to a private place where you won't be overheard and let your emotions take over. Throw old crockery at a wall or hit a heavy bag as you shout curses at whatever has aroused your anger. Play a sad song and sob out loud over the loss of something or someone you loved. Continue this for at least ten minutes—half an hour would be even better.

During the worst periods of my own life, I could spend hours grieving or fussing. However, I benefited greatly from the advice of a therapist who told me not to plunge into the darkness for more than about an hour and a half per day. If you find yourself nearing the hour-and-a-half mark, imagine packing your pain and anger in a Tupperware container, opening a cupboard in your mind, and tidily packing the feelings away. They will be there tomorrow, when your time to express your unhappiness comes around again. This strategy is what one psychologist calls "denial with a little d." It will keep you from getting altogether lost in emotional suffering and allow you to continue feeding your kids, doing your job, and basically living a normal life.

Finally, *if you cannot stop expressing emotional pain, or if you can't feel any emotion at all, the Joy Diet requires that you enter therapy, now.* I'm as serious as a plane crash. There is no such thing as a healthy human being who lacks all feeling, or who is naturally in constant anguish. The total absence or uncontrollable flood of emotion (which are more similar than you might think) means you are drowning in psychological pain too difficult to cope with on your own. You need and deserve professional help, and you must get it.

All of these laughter alternatives, including professional counseling, are temporary measures designed to return you to a place where you laugh often, naturally, and irrepressibly. After you've fully felt and expressed painful emotions, you will find that laughter shows up more and more often in their place. I can't tell you how many times I've sat with grim-faced clients until they felt safe enough to curse or weep, and watched them brighten into genuine, easy laughter almost immediately thereafter. Wherever you are when you begin the Joy Diet, you will eventually get to the point where laughter takes and retains a permanent position of prominence in your daily behavior. Then you can launch into the following strategies along with other Joy Dieters.

Laughter Step 1: Assess Your Innate Laughter Tendencies (Both Quantity and Quality)

When you embark on Menu Item #8, spend a couple of days simply observing your own laughter. Carry a notebook and make a hatchmark every time you chuckle, or use a tally counter (available at any office supply store) as my editor and I did. If you're a natural-born laugher, you may well find that you're already fulfilling the Joy Diet laughter requirements. I suggest that you consider changing your minimum LPD to a hundred laughs or more. Thirty per day is a minimum; the sky's the limit.

Just as important as knowing your numeric laughter rate is noticing what types of stimuli make you laugh. Do you guffaw uncontrollably after saying things like "Hey, how have you been?" or "Do you have a rubber band?" Are ridiculous hairstyles, pratfalls, or other people's misfortunes your prime laughter triggers? Do you like being tickled by scientists? Answering questions like these will help you fulfill Menu Item #8 without wasting time on things you don't find amusing or delightful. You may also want to specify whether you like your humor light, dark, or somewhere in between, so that you can gravitate immediately toward things that will make you laugh most readily. If you're not sure where your humor preferences lie, consider the following three jokes, which I think fall at the light, medium-gray, and dark points on the humor scale. See if any of them appeals to you more than the others.

The first joke comes from a physician who, according to a published study, uses humor to jolly his patients. It goes like this:

EXAMPLE OF A LIGHT JOKE

QUESTION: What's a cold war?
ANSWER: A snowball fight.

I find this about as funny as watching fruit rot, but apparently, certain medical patients think it's just a hoot. These folks might well be offended by the following, somewhat darker quip, which won a 2002 competition to see what joke Americans found most amusing.

EXAMPLE OF A SOMEWHAT DARKER JOKE
(AN AMERICAN FAVORITE)

Two roommates meet on the first day of classes. One of them is a prep-school blueblood, the other a small-town public school grad.

"So," says the small-town girl, "where you from?"

The preppie regards her coldly, then says, "From a place where we know better than to end our sentences with prepositions."

"Ah," the small-town girl replies. "So, where you from, bitch?"

The fact that this joke appealed so much to Americans probably reveals that typical U.S. citizens reach the limits of their comfort zones when considering socially embarrassing situations, such as getting caught using bad grammar, or swearing mildly at a stranger. Other cultures, apparently, are struggling with much darker eventualities. Here is the joke that was found most humorous in several countries other than the United States.

EXAMPLE OF A STILL DARKER JOKE (AN UN-AMERICAN FAVORITE)

Two friends from New Jersey, Bob and Fred, are out in the woods hunting. Suddenly Bob clutches his chest, falls to the ground, flops around for a minute, then goes limp and still.

Horrified, Fred grabs his cell phone and calls 911. When the emergency operator answers, he shouts, "Oh, my God! You've got to help me! Bob died! He had a heart attack and *died!* What should I do?"

"Sir, try to stay calm," says the operator. "I can help. The first thing we have to do is make absolutely sure your friend is really dead."

"All right, just a minute," says Fred. The operator hears a pause, then a single gunshot. Then Fred picks up the phone again and says, "Okay, now what?"

Some of my friends didn't even get this joke, and of those who did, several found it too dark to be funny, although they naturally appreciated the gratuitous New Jersey slam. I like it a lot, but I think we have already established that I am seriously mentally ill. In fact, I am amused by jokes much darker than the preceding one, things I won't even include here for fear of reprisal from upstanding citizens or Republicans. Anyway, it doesn't matter what kind of humor floats your boat, as long as you identify it and feed it to your brain in large, frequent doses.

This means avoiding people and media items (magazine articles, comic books, movies, TV shows) that favor a humor style you dislike, and unabashedly pursuing those that are on your wavelength. When my client Tandy appears too sober, I recommend that she read the "Laughter Is the Best Medicine" page in the most recent *Reader's Digest*. That simply doesn't cut it for me; when I'm running short on laughs, I seek out the people I can rely on to tell jokes that are fundamentally sick and wrong. I also take the following steps, any or all of which you might use if your laughter quota is shy of the Joy Diet mark.

Laughter Step 2: Expose Yourself to Comedy

You may have heard of Norman Cousins, an essayist whose book *Anatomy of an Illness* recounted his recovery from a supposedly incurable spine disease. Cousins decided to take the whole "laughter as medicine" thing literally. He treated his disease by locking himself in a hotel room and watching Marx Brothers movies for several hours every day. According to Cousins, his pain tolerance increased dramatically after he'd been laughing for ten minutes, and if he laughed for three hours in the morning, the rest of his day would be virtually pain-free. Cousins believed that his comedy-fest ultimately broke the grip of the disease.

Though I am most definitely *not* suggesting that you substitute the Marx Brothers for medical care, it never hurts to supplement regular medical care by following Cousins's example, spending some time each day deliberately seeking and enjoying comedy. Here are a few ways you might go about it.

COMEDY SOURCES

1. Browse the "humor" section at your local bookstore. (Bookstores are better in this respect than libraries, because few really silly books are deemed worthy of inclusion in literary collections.)

2. Make sure you never miss your favorite funny television program. Schedule it in your planner. Fit other obligations around it. Show some discipline. If you absolutely insist on having a life outside TV, tape or TiVo comedies until you come to your senses.

3. Read e-mailed jokes *that come from your funniest friends*. Be careful with this one. If you open every "funny" message that floats through your modem, you may destroy your sense of humor, if not your entire mind.

4. Bookmark your favorite funny websites. Then check them daily. Find links to your favorite cartoons ("Dilbert"? "Cathy"? "Classic Peanuts"?). Check out the "Pretty Good Jokes" on Prairie Home Companion's website at *www.phc.mpr.org*. See if anything on *www.theonion.com, www.brunching.com*, or *www.modernhumorist.com* is your cup of tea.

5. Go to comedy clubs, even if they are only the pathetic remnants of the 1980s standup boom. Seeing comedians in person creates more comic energy than watching them on screen.

6. Read movie reviews, and attend films that are labeled funny by several major newspapers. Don't waste your time going to a

Continued

movie if the only positive reviews come from a late-night college radio program broadcast out of rural Wyoming.

7. Rent videos or DVDs of classic comedies from the past. You might want to look up the American Film Critics' list of "the hundred funniest movies ever made." I don't agree with all their selections, and I think they omitted some classics, but this list can certainly get you going.

Laughter Step 3: Hang Out with Laughers

You may notice that you laugh more when you're in a crowded theater than when you're home watching a videotape on your own. That's because laughter, like the tendency to yawn or panic, boasts a high level of "social contagion." Just hearing someone else snorting and gasping primes us to see things from a humorous angle. This is why situation comedies have piped-in laugh tracks, or live audiences primed to respond to flashing "laugh" signs. Some television studios actually pay people with hearty laughs to sit in their audiences and bellow hysterically at every wisp of a joke. You should follow their lead by hanging out with people who laugh easily.

Some of my Joy Diet testers reported very low levels of laughter when they spent time alone, but they could zoom way past the minimum thirty in just a few minutes spent with other people. If you're one of those people who never laughs alone, then in my opinion, falling short of thirty laughs a day means you're not spending enough time in a social context. Make the phone calls. Meet a buddy for coffee. Go to a theater where the crowd is primed to laugh. Do whatever it takes to get your LPD quota up to at least thirty.

Almost all my friends laugh a lot when they're around me, probably because of my hairstyle. On the other hand, these people seem to laugh at pretty much everyone and everything. I appear to gravitate to Frequent Laughers, and I've found that their company is better than prescription antidepressants. I've been collecting these people for years, so I have several high-quality laughter sources available. If you haven't put as much time into your own collection, I urge you to begin: Notice how often the people in your life laugh. Notice how often you laugh when you're talking to them. Keep a mental list of the folks who amuse you most. Memorize their phone numbers. Connect with them at stressful moments when you can't think of anything laughable about your situation, and let them find the funny parts for you. (By the way, these friends should form part of the audience for Laughter Step 6.)

Laughter Step 4: Use Mechanical Stimulation (Stop Smirking; It's a Very Enjoyable Habit)

If you don't know any frequent laughers, audiotapes of guffawing strangers will do almost as well. When I was teaching in business school, I used to break the ice on the first day of class every semester by playing a tape of a working session by writer/actors Mike Nichols and Elaine May. At one point in the tape, Nichols and May break character and dissolve into helpless laughter that goes on for at least five minutes. Even my most stone-faced graduate students couldn't sit through this without starting to chuckle. Playing the tape was like putting sourdough starter in a lump of bread dough; the students performed well and seemed to feel comfortable laughing at me for the entire semester.

You can order the Nichols/May tape (*Mike Nichols and Elaine May in Retrospect*) from a real-space or online music store. If you're really serious about Menu Item #8, order a tape called *The Laughter Album* from the Oxford-based Happiness Project (address orders to Happiness Project, Elms Court, Chapel Way, Oxford, England, OX2 0LP). On this tape, you will hear people laughing. That's all. I know it doesn't sound funny, but if this tape doesn't make you laugh too, you can be declared legally dead in most states.

Laughter Step 5: Laugh for No Reason

If you've mastered all the preceding techniques, you may be ready to take on the ultimate Menu Item #8 challenge: laughing without any discernible cause. During my Joy Diet research, I was startled to learn that there is a legitimate system of yoga (like Hatha or Kundalini) that focuses almost completely on laughter. It's called—I swear on my grandmother this is true—the "Ho-Ho-Ha-Ha-Ha" method. According to the literature, practitioners start this yogic strategy by learning how to laugh for at least a minute with no provocation whatsoever. They also gather and "participate in group laughter every day for 15 to 20 minutes without having to resort to jokes." According to one Ho-Ho-Ha-Ha-Ha teacher, "the practice of daily, unreasonable laughter can become a habit, like brushing your teeth." (Or, perhaps, like fiddling with the string fasteners of the restraining devices the attendants make you wear at night.)

I couldn't find a local Ho-Ho-Ha-Ha-Ha teacher near my home, but I did go so far as to try the techniques recommended on the always-handy Internet. The best I can say for my progress is that at least I have the humility appropriate for my complete lack of talent. I managed only a weak, self-conscious smile, though I did experience a tiny pang of amusement at my own pathetic performance—but then, that amusement had a cause, and the goal is to laugh without one. I tip my hat to those of you who travel the road of laughter unsullied by amusement. If you get the hang of it, will you teach me? Until then, I think it's best for everyone that I continue to rely on drugs.

Laughter Step 6: Laugh at Yourself

All these methods of increasing your LPD are just to get you warmed up for Menu Item #8's pièce de résistance: laughing at yourself. Long ago, I noticed that of all the clients I coached, the most intransigently "stuck" were those who never found anything humorous about their own shortcomings or problems. On the other hand, clients who systematically laughed at themselves, especially in frightening or discouraging circumstances, seemed to push past almost any obstacle to reach their goals. Whenever you feel stuck, laughing at yourself is just the thing to un-stick you. If you're not used to this, there are a couple of ways you might go about it.

The first technique, which you should use if you're a beginner at self-mockery, is simply to violate your usual behavioral rules by acting silly. I like the suggestions offered by an article in the *London Daily Telegraph,* a respectable newspaper in a country known for its love of protocol. After noting the benefits of laughing at oneself, the article suggests that readers gather with friends or family, then "find a word that makes you laugh, and repeat it to each other in silly voices. [Then] walk around the room, trying to impersonate different emotional states: the angry walk, the grumpy walk or the happy walk." I'm sure Queen Elizabeth and Prince Charles use this method on a regular basis, whether they're hosting a state dinner or just spending a little quality time together. I hope the prince is careful when he's wearing one of his kilts.

Speaking of kilts, I've always found that dressing up is a fine way to add silliness to your schedule. My family's annual Winter Solstice celebration is immeasurably enhanced by donning the silliest Viking helmets we can find, including some with built-in hair braids and horns large enough to bedeck a prairie bull. Wearing one of these saves a great deal of humor-directed labor, because you don't have to do anything else to look silly; the more serious you act, the sillier you become. In fact, if you happen to be Tom Brokaw, I challenge you to (just once) do the news in a major hair-braid Viking helmet without comment or explanation. You could create a landmark moment in television journalism, improving millions of people's mood, health, and mental fitness while you're at it.

If you have a favorite form of silliness—say, acting out old Monty Python routines, imitating your iguana, reading (better yet, drawing) cartoons, planning witty things to say to your friends, or simply remembering funny experiences until you feel the tickle factor all over again, give yourself lots of permission to roll around in this behavior. I seem to be unable to keep myself from doing this, and though it looks like an utter waste of time, I believe it has increased my quality of life to an immeasurable degree.

For instance, even during the most hectic times of my life, for no reason except pure silliness, certain friends and I (sometimes together, sometimes on our own, but with the intention of sharing later) would spend hours cutting out odd-looking photographs and vaguely droll magazine headlines, then mixing and matching different words and pictures until one particular combination made us laugh. We'd glue these to a blank piece of paper, then add the page to others, forming what we called, with dazzling originality, a "fun book." I still laugh every time I open one of these books and see, for instance, a picture of a zaftig, tired-looking, middle-aged grandma that bears the caption "The Colorless, Odorless Killer: In Cold Pursuit," or a photo of Chinese veterinarians artificially inseminating a panda, underscored by the words "I Almost Died at the Hands of a Maniac," or the image of a woman with a small pig in her arms and a wild grin on her face, with the headline "Lonely Too Long." Okay, so you have to be there. But try this yourself, and you'll see how much you can enjoy your own absolutely pointless wit.

You should definitely try simple silliness before moving on to the next self-mockery technique, which I consider the most powerful form of Menu Item #8. Like most of the Joy Diet components, it is psychologically difficult, but procedurally quite simple. All you have to do is describe, with complete honesty, an aspect of your life where you feel stuck, frustrated, confused, or uncertain. Talking about these subjects can take you to the edge of the zone where you lose your self-assurance. This will allow you to expand your confidence and make your world bigger.

Old European maps used to show the edges of territory that had been explored by Westerners, then label the unexplored areas with the phrase "Here be dragons." This is how you will feel when you set out to laugh at your own insecurities. You're about to travel to places you'd rather avoid, and it will require some daring. What may surprise you is that the "dragons" in this undiscovered country can be made ridiculous, and this gives you power over them. By allowing your problems to slay you, you can slay them.

So, let's get started. In the following space, list a few frustrating issues that have kept you from accomplishing some of your cherished goals. Maybe you hate your job but don't dare quit. Maybe your mother manipulates you into doing whatever she wants, instead of living the life your heart desires. Many people are embarrassed about some aspect of their personal appearance, although I'm sure this is not true in your case. See if you can think of five issues that are blockading the way to your ideal life.

OBSTACLE ISSUES

1. _____

2. _____

3. _____

4. _____

5. _____

Now, get together with your funniest friends, or, if that's not convenient, imagine that you're sitting with them. While you're at it, you may also want to pretend that you've been transformed into your favorite comedian. Did you ever notice that people often sing better when they're imitating a professional musician? By the same token, most of us become funnier when we impersonate someone who makes us laugh. Standing on the shoulders of comedy giants allows us to see things more whimsically until we develop our own comedic style. If you're just setting out to laugh at yourself, start by reading, hearing, or watching the work of funny people. Apply their perspective to descriptions of your own issues.

Now the stage is set, the audience is in place, and it's time to do some storytelling. You're going to describe your problems and the way you feel about them openly and honestly, without pulling any punches. Conventional wisdom dictates that we should minimize the severity of our problems, pretend we're not as upset about them as we really are, and refuse to discuss things that cause shame or embarrassment. Well, while you're practicing Menu Item #8, I want you to do exactly the opposite. Describe the very worst aspects of your situation. Give the gory details. Express your most horrified reactions. Exaggerate. If there's something humiliating in your situation, something you hope no one will ever know, go there. Talk about it. Remember, the more the subject matter is blocking you, the more you should rant about it. You'll find that the more you push yourself to express the worst-case scenarios, the more ridiculous they'll begin to sound.

Here is a list of questions that might help you address your frustrating issues in this manner. I'll use them on an example from my own life, right at this moment, to show how the process can work.

INTO THE REALM OF DRAGONS: TELLING IT LIKE IT IS (AND THEN SOME)

Q: What is the most upsetting issue pressing on your mind right now?

A: This manuscript is really, really late, and I am writing really, really slowly.

Q: What is your worst fear about this situation?

A: I'll never finish this book, at least not in the present century.

Continued

Q: Can you think of an outcome that's even scarier? Go on, be creative.

A: I won't be able to return the advance money, because I've already spent it, and I'll go deeply in debt to loan sharks, who are the only lenders willing to work with sluggish, dissolute, shiftless authors like me.

Q: And then?

A: I'll become an impoverished fast-food restaurant attendant, but I'll only be able to work for a few months before the job destroys my health, making me so tired that I'll cause an enormous grease fire that will permanently disfigure me. I'll be unable to get another job because of the constant pain and my ghastly appearance. To help pay the mortgage, my children will drop out of school, sell themselves into prostitution, and contract every STD known to medicine. We will all die on the street and be eaten by rats and mice, who will chuckle in a sinister, mocking fashion the entire time, though the sound they make will be so different from us that it will be hard to directly equate it with human laughter.

Q: Very good. Now, what is particularly embarrassing about your problem? Is there anything you'd like to hide?

A: I haven't answered the phone for six weeks, because I'm afraid it will be either my editor or my agent, both of whom are loving and gracious and hate being forced to nag me, which makes me feel so guilty I'd like to . . .

Q: To what?

A: I haven't decided, but I'm thinking of giving alcoholism a try.

Q: Fine. Is there anything even more embarrassing you'd like to share?

A: When I do answer the phone, I fake a Croatian accent and tell callers I am profoundly deaf. But I think they can tell it's me.

Q: I think so. Now, what about this issue makes you angry?

A: My computers keep crashing. This is my third desktop setup in two books.

Q: What does your anger make you want to do?

A: I want to bitch-slap every employee in IBM's Tech Support department, then keep them all on "hold" for twenty-five years to life.

I think you can see where this is going. Remember Milarepa, the Tibetan sage who lay down in a demon's mouth to vanquish it? Talking about your frustrations not only openly, but excessively, pursuing them to their most comically unlikely outcomes in a deliberate attempt to make others laugh, pulls out their fangs and claws. Remember that your goal is entertainment, not pity—there's nothing *less* funny than begging for sympathy—then go ahead and rant. The more you stride right straight at your problems by telling the truth about your fear, frustration, anger, and even sadness, the more the dragons will retreat, and the bigger your world will become.

There is no upper limit to the recommended Joy Diet LPD. On a good day, you may find that you can get yours up into the hundreds. But even on the not-so-good days, the days when everything goes wrong and the world is ashes in your mouth, finding a way to laugh thirty times can open you to new ways of coping with your distress. It will enhance every good thing you do on the Joy Diet, the way a filter can brighten a photograph. True, as you become more and more prone to laughter, some people will disapprove. They'll look at you askance, purse their narrow lips, and in various other ways suggest that you should return to a world dominated by fear. They may accuse you of childishness. They'll be right. If you keep heading in this direction, you may well end up laughing as much as you did when you were little and adventurous and continually surprised by joy. Personally, that's a risk I'm prepared to take.

MENU ITEM #8: LAUGHTER

MINIMUM DAILY REQUIREMENTS

1. Assess your innate laughter tendencies. Observe yourself to see whether you're meeting the thirty LPD minimum. Note the quality and darkness of your preferred humor.

2. Expose yourself to comedy. You can do this either live or through entertainment-media sources.

3. Hang out with laughers. Make a list of Frequent Laughers you know. Memorize their numbers.

4. Use mechanical stimulation. Recordings of nothing but laughter sound boring, but they're not.

5. Learn to laugh for no reason. There is an entire branch of yoga devoted to helping with this.

6. Laugh at yourself. Identify the issues that make you most uncomfortable. Set the stage by taking the position of a comic addressing an audience. Exaggerate the pain.

CONNECTION

·

EVERY DAY, USE JOY DIET SKILLS 1 THROUGH 5 (DOING NOTHING, TELLING THE TRUTH, IDENTIFYING YOUR HEART'S DESIRES, USING YOUR CREATIVITY, AND TAKING A RISK) IN AT LEAST ONE INTERACTION WITH A PERSON WHO IS IMPORTANT IN YOUR LIFE.

IF YOU ARE PLAYING BY THE RULES OF THE JOY DIET, as I am *sure* you are, you will already have smoothly incorporated Menu Items #1 through #8 into your daily behavioral routine. You'll have them all down pat by now, be using them as fluently and as readily as your mother tongue.

No?

Okay, then, all I'm asking is, for God's sake, try to get a decent handle on the previous menu items before you attempt to proceed to #9. The elements of the Diet are arranged so that by the time you get to this step, you'll have been practicing things like nothing-doing and telling the truth for several weeks. You'll need these skills to master Menu Item #9, and trust me, this is something you want to do. It can bring you more wonderful and unexpected kinds of joy than any other item on the Diet. It's a ticket out of the deepest kinds of despair, the balm to cool your hottest anger, the security harness that will help you turn your worst fears into courage and confidence. That's not because this menu item itself is particularly dazzling, but because it creates, sustains, and strengthens your link to something that can be: other people.

Adding this menu item to your life is easy if you've mastered earlier steps, especially Menu Items #1 through #5. All you have to do to create powerful, healing, enlightening relationships is apply the first five Joy Diet techniques to an interaction with another human being. Do this at least once every day. It won't take a bit more time than you'd spend interacting any other way. The person you choose to connect with in this Joy Diet way might be a friend, family member, or spouse/partner. It could also be anyone you work with: your boss, a subordinate, a coworker, customer, or client.

You may recall that Menu Item #7, though it can be applied to personal relationships, is mainly targeted to affect your life's work. Menu Item #9, by contrast, is very good for your career, but will play out mainly in personal relationships. This chapter describes how you can incorporate Menu Item #9 and its many benefits into your life as a whole.

Master Doing Nothing, Telling Yourself the Truth, Identifying Your Heart's Desires, and Daring to Risk

Suppose you took just one tennis lesson, then went out to play a match against an experienced opponent. Every time the ball headed your way, you'd have a dozen things to think about: whether to use a forehand or backhand grip, how to place your feet correctly, how to create a decent backswing, whether it was a mistake to wear a halter unitard—forget it, that ball's long gone. Well, the menu items on the Joy Diet are like tennis fundamentals, or for that matter, any other learned behavior. If you practice them consistently, they gradually become smoother, more efficient, and more automatic. To really see how Menu Item #9 can work, you need to internalize the first five Joy Diet items until they become familiar.

I tend to nurture the delusional conviction that I can learn any skill by reading about it. I churn through books like this in a single sitting, thinking, "Yeah, yeah, I get it—I don't need to do your damn exercises." If you share this tendency, I must reiterate that the ability to slide into nothingness, to tell and recognize the bare-bones truth, to locate and define your heart's desires, to solve problems creatively, and to consistently take small, graduated risks are very different in action than in description.

After years of doing nothing as often as possible, for example, I can now achieve a state of calm, often verging on torpor, in situations that once would have unhinged me entirely. My years of focusing on my best guess at the truth have helped me recognize my lies and drag my secrets into the light more quickly. My heart's desires, which used to elude my conscious mind for years on end, barely even bother to hide from me nowadays. I tend to get creative rather than giving up when I run into problems. And my determination to take risks has solidified as I benefit from doing it. What I'm saying is, practice, practice, practice. You need to have these skills built in, because you're about to hit center court and play a match with another human being. Using your Joy Diet skills in the context of a relationship will create a whole new set of challenges, and you need the fundamentals in place.

Relationship Dynamics:
One Plus One Equals Three

My favorite art professor used to teach his students that in drawing, one plus one always equals three. This is because when you draw two figures on a piece of paper, there are three visual images that will catch the viewer's eyes: the two things you've drawn, and the blank space between them. You may have seen the faces/vases optical trick, where two profiles drawn opposite each other form the image of a chalice in the space between them. One face plus one face equals two faces and one vase.

In human relationships, as well as art, one plus one equals three. Every pairing of two different people forms a unique synergy, an emotional reality that could not exist without both parties and cannot be duplicated by any other combination. There is always a you, a me, and an us. It is this curious third element—the unique "us" formed by every "you" and "me"—that allows human beings to maintain emotional well-being.

Saying that we are social creatures doesn't begin to describe how vital connection is to every single one of us. A person forced into solitary confinement suffers unimaginably, even with enough food and shelter to last until doomsday. Babies who aren't held may die; babies who never have an adult gaze lovingly into their eyes may grow up with severe mental illness. Psychologist Judith Hermann, an expert in the study of trauma, writes that while the unit of human physical survival is one, the unit of psychological survival is two. Without someone to connect with, we quite simply can't go on. Not any of us.

You'll hear a lot about emotional connection if you listen to popular music, watch television, or go to the movies. American culture is particularly obsessed with connection in the form of romantic love. I've had many clients who thought that all their problems—unhappiness, lack of motivation, job failure, toe fungus—would magically disappear once the right person fell in love with them. As far as I could tell, they were waiting for this great event without making the slightest attempt to solve these problems themselves, or to become the sort of person anyone would fall in love with. But the truth is that romantic love isn't a panacea, and that any connection between any two people, not just lovers, changes the world.

For example, I know one woman who survived an emotionally barren childhood on the strength of one fleeting encounter with a person whose name she never knew. "I was about four," Chloe recalls, "and my father had taken me to his office for some reason. There was a secretary there who reacted to me in a way I'd never experienced. Her whole being seemed to light up when she saw me. I think she was just one of those people who love all children. While my dad went into his office, this woman came over to me and crouched down, so our eyes were level. I can't recall what she said. But while she talked, she looked straight into my eyes. I couldn't remember anyone ever doing that before. And I remember feeling, all the way through my body, 'She *sees* me!'"

Chloe can't tell this story without crying. Much later, she would go searching for that sense of being seen, and because she knew what to look for, she would eventually find it. She never encountered the secretary again. But that moment of connection was the slim line that kept Chloe tied to humanity for much of her life. If you become skilled at the art of connection, I can't even guess how many lives you may transform. I only know that one of them will be your own.

Hidden Disconnection

My client Dave is a professional athlete who's accustomed to hearing tens of thousands of fans cheering his name. Yet, right in the middle of a game, with this hurricane of adulation roaring around him, he often feels desperately lonely. Hillary is a popular entertainer who just got married to a great guy. They spend every day together (and they look sensational!), but both say they feel more isolated than before they married. Sally is a minister, surrounded by adoring congregants who tell her their deepest thoughts, yet she feels so alone that she's beginning to question her faith in both God and the human race. Joe is a born leader; his employees would literally spend their lives following him. But he, too, is dogged by a terrible loneliness. I could give you literally hundreds of other examples of successful, well-loved people whose central problem is a feeling of isolation.

The problem is that just having relationships, even being surrounded by huge crowds of people who love you, isn't the same as really connecting, heart to heart. The four people I've just described (five, if you count Hillary's husband) all have a habit of actually avoiding deep, genuine emotional connection. Why? Because to connect with another human being is incredibly risky. As soon as you make genuine contact with another person, there are two things intimately connected to you that are not under your control: the other person, and the relationship you now share. That means you become vulnerable to all sorts of potentially devastating outcomes: rejection, obligation, heartbreak, loss.

To people who have been hurt by any previous painful relationship, from childhood on (and by this I mean everybody), such vulnerability is terrifying. Most of us don't articulate the fear that comes with connecting to another; instead, we try desperately to eliminate this fear by controlling the situation. One control mechanism is simply to refuse any form of intimacy. The more popular method is to try to control the people who matter to us—whether they're lovers, children, employees, or what have you—so that they can never leave, hurt, or dominate us.

The methods we use in our efforts to control others are almost infinite. Many of them don't overtly look like control at all. For instance, my favorite form of interpersonal control is people-pleasing. I will give myself literal, physical hernias trying to make people happy, purely so that I won't have to tolerate the horrible possibility that they might not like me. I act this way even toward people I detest. I'm telling you, it's very, very annoying. Of course, on occasion I can resort to other control techniques, such as manipulation, withholding information, and the occasional old-fashioned tantrum. You probably have your own favorites: righteous indignation, overt helplessness, shaming, persuasion, violence, seductiveness, cold indifference, lying . . . we could go on all day, couldn't we?

If you're the high achiever I'm guessing you are, you may spend virtually all your time trying to buy risk-free love through spectacular success. Dave, my professional-athlete client, always believed that if he could make it to the top in his sport, he'd finally feel acceptable, sure that others would never reject him. Hillary felt the same way about being an entertainer, and about the bonds of holy matrimony—once a guy put a ring on her finger, she figured, he *couldn't* hurt or abandon her. Sally went into the ministry because she thought being needed in people's spiritual lives was a guarantee of unconditional love. Joe, the dynamic company president, thought that if he formed a business that gave other people a livelihood, he could relax and trust their connection to him. These people went to astonishing extremes trying to nail down a human connection without taking any chance of getting hurt.

It can't be done.

What can be done, however, is to form deep, nourishing emotional connections that will keep you feeling sane and blessed no matter what the other person chooses to do. You accomplish this by loving unconditionally and unilaterally. But doesn't this strategy virtually guarantee you'll get hurt? No, silly. It doesn't virtually guarantee that you'll be wounded. It *absolutely* guarantees it. Some of the people you connect with will be cruel. Some will be self-destructive. Some of them will die before you do. It's going to be just awful. But as long as you never react by cutting off your willingness to love, you will always—*always*—emerge from these situations with more capacity for joy than you took into them. You will win emotional security neither by finding some infallible person to love, nor by controlling people who are fallible, but by constantly using your ability to connect. Give me a fish, I eat for a day; teach me to fish, I eat for a lifetime. So. Let's go fishing.

Using Your Joy Diet Skills to Form Connections

The Hawthorne Effect is named after a match factory in Hawthorne, Massachusetts, where efficiency experts once decided to see how much the lighting inside the plant affected the workers' output. It seemed obvious that the more light the workers had, the better they'd perform. So researchers were startled when on the first day of their study, they dimmed the lights—and the workers' productivity increased! Dramatically! The next day the researchers dimmed the lights even more, and sure enough, the workers did even better. The efficiency experts kept making the place darker and darker until the factory workers were trying to function in the same level of light they'd get from the moon, at which point their productivity finally slackened.

Why did this happen? Well, it turned out that the lighting had virtually nothing to do with the Hawthorne workers' sudden increase in productivity. The reason they'd upped their output was simply that *they knew they were being watched*. The psychological impact of another person's presence—any other person's presence—is incredibly strong, so strong it can overwhelm almost every other factor in our environment.

We're all susceptible to various versions of the Hawthorne Effect. No matter how functional we are, being in the presence of any new person is a whole new ball game. There are some folks around whom we feel relaxed and easy, others who set our teeth on edge to an embarrassing degree. I have certain clients who fill me with energy and others who suck the strength out of me like lampreys. My job, in my office as in any other setting, is to remain grounded in my own truth and sense of self, even as I let myself experience the emotional energy created by the other person's presence. The best way to accomplish this is to do nothing—and you know I mean really nothing.

Connection Step 1: Learn to Reach the Place of Peace While with Another Person

If you think doing nothing is hard when you're by yourself, try it with another person staring at you. I do this during every session I spend with a client, and each time, it makes me incredibly nervous. I start doing nothing a few minutes prior to the client's arrival, just to prime the pump. Then, when the person is sitting across from me, I sustain my nothing-doing behavior: I keep breathing deeply and noticing my own thoughts when they arise, even while I'm listening to the client. In accordance with my overall life goal (do nothing, get paid), I try to stay centered throughout the session, no matter what the client says or does. I always fail. My attention repeatedly rollicks off, trying to fix or impress or convince or (above all) please the client. That's okay. What matters is that I notice when I've lost my connection to the great stillness, and I bring my attention back.

I'm not sure what effect this has on my clients, but it certainly does a number on me. I have found that it is impossible to truly do nothing while interacting with another person and not fall in love with them. No, I don't follow my clients home to lurk in their shrubbery with a zoom-lens camera and a jar of Ben-Gay. But while they're in my office, and when I'm successfully doing nothing, I see in each of them a being of such breathtaking beauty and value that I can hardly stand it. This is true even of people I don't like—at least not with the small mind I use in daily living. Some clients seem to appreciate my advice, some don't. Some will come back, some won't. Sometimes I think I help, and sometimes I do such a terrible job it makes me cringe for years afterward. None of that changes the fact that invariably, by watching each person from a place of inner stillness, my life is deepened and enriched.

The same thing happens when you consider the people you love from a position of centered nothing-doing. When you're doing nothing, caring for your screaming toddler creates only empathy for what it's like to be a very ambitious person in a very small body. If you do nothing while looking across a restaurant table at a friend, you may feel such love it will split you in half. Go to the great silence when you're in bed with your heartthrob, and you'll see that all the greatest songs and paintings and poems about romantic love are pathetic under-statements. The Place of Peace is a place of pure love, and from there, you cannot help but form and strengthen connections with the people in your life.

When you first begin working on Menu Item #9, I suggest you focus on strangers. Sit in a café, or airport, and use what-ever nothing-doing technique works best for you. See what happens when you look out from nothing at that woman with the ridiculous Botox overdose, the man whose eyes drop when the waitress speaks to him. Breathe, be still, and watch your thoughts. The deeper you go into silent awareness, the more you will see these people's hearts.

Next, use nothing-doing during idle conversations with friends or colleagues. Become still just for a moment, when there's a lull. You'll find that instead of distracting you, doing nothing allows you to perceive and understand your compan-ion more clearly. I've had many clients tell me that they become much more intuitive, much more able to "read" people, when they practice this behavior.

Your next step is to do nothing when you're with people you love. This will just knock you right over. When I do this practice regularly, I walk around feeling as though I'm made of warm wax, constantly stretching and softening in order to con-tain a sweetness that never seems to stop getting bigger. Try doing nothing when you're angry, grief-stricken, bored, or anxious; you'll find that you react to your loved ones less nega-tively. You'll feel less desire to control your significant others, and more desire to simply be present with them—which is probably all they want from you.

The downside of this whole procedure is that it really will cause you to love the people you interact with unconditionally, whether or not they decide to misbehave, tell lies, smoke crack, dump you like a sack of slag, or drive like a maniac and die in a car crash. But if you remain in your Place of Peace even as your heart breaks, you'll find that it always breaks open. Keep doing nothing, naming your sorrow and rage and anguish as they surge through you, and they leave much more quickly than they would if you fought not to experience them. You'll learn much more from the process, too, so that the next time you meet someone who fits the dysfunctional profile you always found irresistible, you'll resist it without even thinking. An open heart is like a prospector's pan; it allows all the useless dross to drift away, and when the pain is gone, whatever pure gold there was to be had in the relationship remains. You get to keep that, forever, as long as you are willing to simply remain present.

Cultivating nothing-doing while interacting with others is the basis of connection because it situates you in your true self and helps you see the true selves of others. False selves—the attention-grabbing, controlling, fearful sides of our personalities—never really connect, no matter how much affection they feign. Just an instant of true contact, like Chloe's encounter with the secretary, is worth all the unctuous pseudo-friendships you'll ever have. Becoming still will link you with those who are meant to love you. It will also seriously unnerve anyone who is out to get you—but that is not a reason for doing it. That's just a bonus.

Connection Step 2: Learn to Tell Yourself the Truth While Interacting with Someone Else

The great majority of pain you have felt because of relationships, including loneliness over the lack of them, is "dirty pain," a product of your own thinking. If you have learned to tell yourself the truth-and-nothing-but-the-truth, you are already light-years ahead of most people in your ability to form healthy connections with others. I suggest you begin using your Menu Item #2 skills to analyze a relationship you're already in. Choose a person about whom you spend considerable time thinking, brooding, or otherwise perseverating. It could be a loved one or someone you hate more than Spam on toast. It could be a movie star you've never met or a fourth-grade sweetheart you haven't seen since the Bronze Age. All that matters is that you feel connected to this person. We will refer to him or her as You Know Who, or YKW.

Now, at a time when you know you're going to be thinking about YKW anyway, go through the "truth" questions from Menu Item #2, and answer them in regard to this person. Here are the questions, modified slightly to help you think in terms of your relationships. I'll discuss them in the text that follows.

TRUTH QUESTIONS (TO BE ANSWERED IN REGARD TO YOU KNOW WHO)

What am I feeling about this person?

Is there anything about this relationship that hurts?

What is the story I'm telling myself about this person?

Can I be sure my story is true?

Is my story working (helping me feel more clear, sane, and free in this relationship)?

Can I think of another story that might work better?

WHAT AM I FEELING ABOUT THIS PERSON?

Remember to stick to descriptions of your emotions—not thoughts, not explanations, not discussions about what you hope will happen. "I feel that he is a nasty horrible ogre" is a thought. "She should love me more" is a thought. A description of the emotions behind these thoughts might be, "I'm full of rage, disgust, and envy. I feel three years old." Or, "I feel love, humiliation, and frustration." You don't have to justify your feelings, but you don't get to edit them, either. Just feel what you feel.

IS THERE ANYTHING ABOUT THIS RELATIONSHIP THAT HURTS?

At this point, painful elements of the situation that has brought you into contact with YKW will begin to emerge. Occasionally, there will be no hurt to describe. Lucky you! If there is something painful, though, don't be afraid to write it all down. "I think he likes me 'that way,' and it's giving me the creeps" might be one answer. "I loathe her, and she's above me in the corporate hierarchy" is another possibility. By all means, go on. Pour out your frustrations, your disappointments, and your anxieties about the future. But remember, *you are only allowed to record your own thoughts, feelings, and empirical observations.* You can include descriptions of things YKW has done, but since you cannot know for sure what any other person feels, you can't write your suppositions about YKW's feelings as though they were facts.

WHAT IS THE STORY I'M TELLING MYSELF ABOUT THIS PERSON?

Whenever we interact with other people, our brains process the experience in two different ways, handled by two different parts of the brain. On one hand, we take in information through our senses and our analytical minds. On the other, we create a little internal narrative to make sense of what we observe. Without realizing it, we "spin" the evidence, deciding what the other person felt, thought, and intended. It feels as though we're simply observing the truth, but in fact, the story we tell about our interpersonal connections is saturated with internalized biases. Once I was walking into a public building with a coworker when an elderly gentleman opened the door for us. After we'd entered the building, and the man was gone, my coworker and I spoke simultaneously. I said, "What a nice man!" and she said, "What a chauvinist pig!" My story was that the guy was being polite and high-minded. My coworker's was that he saw her as weak and therefore inferior.

I once had a client named Pierre who wanted very much to find the right woman but was terrified of rejection. We were both thrilled when Pierre met Emily, the aerobics instructor of his dreams, and their first three dates went beautifully. Then catastrophe struck, at least from Pierre's perspective: Emily called to say she'd have to take a rain check on their next evening out, because her uncle had died and she had to go out of town for the funeral.

"Pretty obvious what's going on, isn't it?" Pierre said after telling me this.

"Um, well, I guess so," I said. "Her uncle died. She has to go to the funeral."

Pierre snorted derisively. "Oh please. It's my hair. She figured out I'm losing my hair." He was so convinced of this that he was planning to end the relationship.

CAN I BE SURE MY STORY IS TRUE?

I reacted so strongly to Pierre's biased interpretation of his interaction with Emily (I think I laughed out loud for a full minute) that he decided to do a little research before he passed judgment. He found a website for the newspaper in the town where Emily's uncle had supposedly lived and died. Sure enough, they had run a recent obituary for someone with Emily's surname, and the funeral was on the very day she had claimed to be attending it. Pierre's relationship was back on.

Unfortunately, not many of our relationship stories are this easy to disprove. We all carry "hangovers" from our childhoods, assumptions we make about people's motivations and actions that may actually (though not necessarily) apply very well to whoever raised us, but often can't be generalized to anyone else. For example, my mother used to do housework when she was very, very angry. For years, every time I saw someone wash a pan or dust a lampshade, I'd go pale with dread at the fury I was sure lay just beneath their calm exteriors. This kind of assumption can be so deep, so taken-for-granted, that until we articulate our stories, we don't even know we're telling them to ourselves. Articulating these tales explicitly is the beginning of all healthy connection.

IS MY STORY WORKING (HELPING ME FEEL MORE CLEAR, SANE, AND FREE IN THIS RELATIONSHIP)?

If you believe something about another person that is not true, your connection to them will be fraught with misunderstanding and misery. Believing untrue stories causes us to act in ways that make no sense to the people around us, since their real motivations and feelings don't match our beliefs. For example, my client Hillary thought that her husband's calm, reserved manner meant he no longer felt any passion toward her. He, in fact, was holding back his emotions out of humiliation, thinking that her clipped, angry manner toward him meant she wasn't interested in making love. Their stories fed into each other, driving them further and further apart over issues neither had ever discussed with the other.

If a relationship isn't working, whether at home or in the workplace, it's usually because one or both parties is holding on to a belief about the other that isn't true. This may be due to misinterpretation, or it may be that one party is lying or keeping secrets. Both situations create a sense of craziness, of things not making sense. If you feel this way, consider that you may be believing lies—either those you tell yourself, or those someone else is telling you.

CAN I THINK OF ANOTHER STORY THAT MIGHT WORK BETTER?

When we free ourselves from the prisons of untruths and allow ourselves to have a "don't-know mind" in regard to a relationship, we may discover that we already know a great deal more about the truth than we thought. One of my clients, Shari, was dating a wonderful man she loved very much, but something felt off. One day I asked her to simply open her mind and see what she felt was true. She thought for a minute, then said, "Children. He has children, and he doesn't want to leave them." Her boyfriend had never mentioned having a wife or children, but when Shari confronted him, he confessed to having both. He claimed not to love his wife, but refused to divorce her because of the effect it might have on the children.

By the way, I don't think this was a psychic deduction on Shari's part. We pick up extremely subtle signals from each other, to the point where we can often tell a great deal about another person just by trusting an instinctive hunch—but remember, check before you treat such things as Absolute Truth. Don't-know mind is good for a relationship; I-know-everything mind is not.

Connection Step 3: Identify What You Want in the Relationship

Clients often tell me that they are careful not to express their real wants and needs in a relationship. They say this as though it were a virtue. "I would never tell my mother how much I want to move away—it would kill her." "I wish my wife understood how hard it is for me to make as much money as she wants me to, but of course, I'd never say anything about it—she'd just feel guilty." "What I'd really like is for us to get away together. If he loved me, he could see that."

If you are one of these silently wistful wanters, I'd like to say to you what I said to the clients I've just quoted. HELLO! ARE YOU COMPLETELY OUT OF YOUR MIND? How in the world do you expect to get what you want out of a relationship if you never define it? You are responsible for identifying and expressing your heart's desires in every relationship, from your marriage to your daily chat with your office manager. At least in your own mind, spell out exactly what you want in very specific detail. Being able to specify is the key to eliminating the insane expectation that the other person will read your mind and figure out how to meet your desires before you do.

If you're feeling anger, *exactly* what is it you want the other person to do or stop doing? If you're feeling love, do you want to express it? Do you want it to be reciprocated, or will loving from afar meet your needs? If you're feeling sad, realize that this is a response to loss, and that it is your job to grieve until that loss is fully processed. Decide whether you need talk, silent company, or some other form of comfort. If you're feeling fear, have the guts to admit it, and decide what you really want to do anyway.

WHAT DO YOU WANT IN YOUR RELATIONSHIP WITH YKW?

Go ahead, tell it like it is. Use extra paper, if you need. Just be very specific.

_____

_____

_____

_____

_____

_____

Connection Step 4: Risk Openness

I don't recommend that you call YKW this very instant and pour out every thought you've just examined and written down. There really is such a thing as too much information, at least in any given moment. Trust your desires to give you the right advice, not just about what you need in a relationship, but about when and how to share that information. When it's time to be open about something, you'll know, because you'll want to say it. You'll want the other person to know it. You may be terrified of the vulnerability you'll feel when you open up, but desire will urge you to do it anyway. Follow its guidance.

WHAT WOULD YOU SAY TO YKW IF YOU HAD NO FEAR?

It doesn't matter how scared you are; write what your heart wants YKW to hear.

_____

_____

_____

_____

_____

_____

My clients' main regrets never involve risking too much. They regret what they didn't say to a loved one or an enemy, what they didn't ask their parents until it was too late, what they didn't say in public when it could have made a difference. It hurts terribly when you take the risk of openness and the reaction is cruel or dishonest. It hurts more when you stay silent when your heart is urging you to speak. And then there are the times when you take that terrifying plunge, when you dare to be open without any assurance that you'll be well received except the conviction of your desire, and it works. Lord almighty, that's the best rush you're ever going to get.

I once went through a time—my turbulent second pregnancy—when what looked like very bad luck came into my life along with some extraordinary privileges. I experienced things I could only explain as miraculous, and they rocked my world to its foundation. Afterward, I kept these experiences bottled up, thinking that I'd be heavily medicated and locked away if I ever told anyone about them. But I wanted—desperately wanted—to communicate to someone what had happened to me, and how I felt about it. I started by telling a few people, with fear and trembling that was partially substantiated. Some of my friends reacted beautifully; others clearly thought I'd gone a little nuts. I found, to my surprise, that the humiliation I took away from the negative encounters was more than balanced by the sense of connection I got from the positive ones. Even so, I still felt like an oddity in the context of Humanity In General. My true self wanted a broader sense of connection. I finally wrote down my experience as a "novel," thinking that this would be a safe way to open up without, you know, actually opening up. My editor would have none of that—she insisted that I write the book as nonfiction. Again, my desires corroborated her opinion.

I began writing my memoir in a computer document I entitled "Help!" I was absolutely quivering with fear. I began the book with a true story about a stranger who told me she had received a message for me from my (three-year-old, nonverbal) son. The message was, "You will never be hurt as much by being open as you have been hurt by remaining closed." At the time this happened, the message sounded like gibberish to me. But years later, it gave me the tenuous dram of confidence I needed to write down the truth.

Since that book was published I've received several hundred letters and e-mails from readers all over the world. A handful of them had precisely the reaction I once feared from everyone: that I am completely nuts and should see a psychiatrist today, before I hurt someone. But the immense majority of messages are from people more kind, forgiving, understanding, and accepting than I thought possible. Though I don't have time to answer all of them (if you sent one, I did read it; thank you), I feel as though each letter-writer is a kindred spirit, a true friend I would never have known existed if I hadn't taken a little risk that seemed huge to me at the time.

This is just one example of the kind of things that happen when we go into the stillness of our real selves, learn what is truest for us, let ourselves feel what we want to do about it, and risk communicating openly in any relationship. Those four steps forge connections between each of us and the rest of the human race, the precious links that join us to health, to happiness, and to each other. You have the skills. Now, I dare you: Use them.

MENU ITEM #9: CONNECTION
MINIMUM DAILY REQUIREMENTS

Master the first four Joy Diet components: doing nothing, telling yourself the truth, identifying your heart's desires, and daring to risk. Practice these until they become familiar, if not automatic. Don't worry if it takes a while; there's plenty of time.

1. Learn to reach the place of peace while with another person.

2. Learn to tell yourself the truth while interacting with someone else. While thinking about someone who occupies a lot of your mental energy, ask yourself the questions you've learned for seeking your inner truth. These questions, modified to fit relationship issues, are as follows:

What am I feeling about this person?
Is there anything about this relationship that hurts?
What is the story I'm telling myself about this person?
Can I be sure my story is true?
Is my story working (helping me feel more clear, sane, and free in this relationship)?
Can I think of another story that might work better?

3. Identify what you want in the relationship. Be very honest and very specific about your desires. It's your responsibility to state them.

4. Risk openness. When desire prompts you to talk about something in your heart, dare to speak up even if part of you is terrified.

FEASTING

•

HAVE AT LEAST THREE SQUARE FEASTS A DAY. THIS MAY INVOLVE FOOD. THEN AGAIN, IT MAY NOT.

I WAS LIVING IN SINGAPORE AT THE TIME. I'D JUST traveled to the United States to attend my sister's wedding, and now, a week later, I was back in Asia again. My circadian rhythm was thoroughly confused by the double whammy of two massive time-zone changes within ten days, so I was pleased to see that the in-flight magazine for Singapore Airlines contained an article about overcoming jet lag. The key to this process, it said, was scheduling food intake. Travelers were supposed to eat at certain hours, depending on how many time zones they were crossing, and strictly abstain from food the remainder of the day. The article listed "feast/fast" schedules for several different travel itineraries. I eagerly looked up the one that was closest to mine. The chart said something like "feast, fast, feast, fast, fast, feast," as if the author were sending a secret message in some kind of dietetic Morse code. But in my bleary-eyed incoherence, I misread the series of words. I thought the prescription said, "feast, feast, feast, feast, feast, feast."

I remember feeling that telltale signal, a spontaneous smile, ripple through my body. I was authorized for constant feasting! As an American female, I had grown used to thinking that the occasional half-cup of chopped celery was a righteous and appropriate diet. I couldn't recall genuinely feasting since early childhood. The word *feast* brought back memories from my first few Thanksgivings, when I was too young to be diet-conscious: the lovely chaos of sounds, sights, and aromas that swirled around me as my huge family crowded into the kitchen to cook (my seven siblings and I were each assigned to make a certain dish), then sat down at two heavily laden tables to inhale what we'd prepared. My father, a wiry little man, would remind us how to tell when we'd eaten enough: The first sign would be a blinding flash; then, after a few more forkfuls, everything would go black. The feasts of my childhood were loud and funny and obstreperous and wonderful. And I had given them up for lost.

It took only a few seconds, there on the Singapore airliner, for me to realize that I'd misread that jet-lag article. No, I did not have permission to indulge myself in nonstop feasts. I'd only discovered a new form of dietary discipline to impose on my hapless body. I remember sighing with disappointed resignation, but even so, something had changed in me. For the first time in years I had allowed myself to picture living a life full of feasts, and that glimpse was so seductive to my true self that it never completely faded. It took another decade or so before I realized that I not only could, but should, "feast feast feast feast feast feast." Now I try to live that way all the time. I don't mean that I never stop eating. I mean that I constantly remind myself to return to the spirit of feasting, to observe the rituals of festivity. That way, things that might slip by me disguised as "ordinary" experiences become feasts for the appetites, the senses, the mind, the heart.

The Joy Diet recommends that you, too, do a great deal of feasting. Three feasts per day are a minimum, and if you're half trying, you can do more. This will require you to assume a mind-set that is the complement of your "treats" perspective. When you give yourself a treat, the objective is to see the well-meaning, useful animal side of your being, tossing yourself small rewards in order to train your beastly self to do things it might not otherwise attempt. When you set out to have a feast, you focus on your uniquely human capacity to be moved and inspired by situations an animal might not even notice. You can call this aspect of yourself whatever you like: your higher consciousness, your soul, your ability to think symbolically, your spirit. Where a treat offers a small, special, tangible reward, a feast is designed to turn your attention to the sublime aspects of things that may, at first glance, seem quite ordinary.

A treat can become a feast, but it doesn't have to. Conversely, a feast may involve unusual treats, but it doesn't require them. For example, you might give yourself a treat by eating your favorite kind of sandwich for lunch, period. If it occurs to you, you might make this event double as a feast by going through the steps of Menu Item #10, which will turn your conscious attention to the effect your sandwich has on your spirit (for example, creating comfort, enjoyment, and a sense of abundance). Later that day, you may be experiencing something completely usual, such as doing the job you've loved for years, when you get the urge to turn this, too, into a feast. You can do it without any physical deviation from your ordinary routine. The steps for creating a feast involve channeling your attention, not obtaining rewards.

This chapter describes how to organize and run a Joy Diet feast, then suggests a few model feasts you might want to throw for yourself. Once you get going on the project, I'm sure you'll be able to elaborate on these ideas, figuring out new kinds of feasting that work especially well for you.

How to Throw a Feast

The most commonly used meaning of the word *feast,* of course, is a large meal. Breakfast, lunch, high tea, or dinner could certainly serve as your Menu Item #10 on any given day. However, most feasts (as defined by the Joy Diet) won't involve food, and a big bunch o' food won't always qualify as a Joy Diet feast. A compulsive eating binge, for example, is the opposite of a feast. It is isolating and tasteless and sickening; it robs delight from both the senses and the soul. On the other hand, hearing a symphony or gazing at the curve of your lover's left elbow could definitely count as feasts, provided that you pay them the right kind of attention. It is not the presence of food or drink that makes a Joy Diet feast, but a sequence of three elements: celebration, nourishment, and thanks. Let's discuss each of these elements, then talk about how you can combine them to create Menu Item #10.

Feast Step 1: Create a Context of Celebration

Celebration is not just happiness or enthusiasm, it is happiness and enthusiasm concretized in behavior—in particular, some form of ritual. A ritual is a set of behaviors designed to show that your soul (or true self, or symbolic consciousness) finds deep meaning in what you are doing. You can adopt the rituals of your culture or tradition, or you can invent them yourself.

Either way, they direct your attention to the symbolic significance of your actions. "Rites," says Antoine de St. Exupery's fictional fox in *The Little Prince,* "are actions too often neglected. They are what make one day different from the other days, one hour from the others." A ritual, however simple, creates a border around a certain activity the way a frame does around a picture. It sets this activity apart from ordinary life in a way that emphasizes beauty and pleasure, ensuring that those who participate in it become more aware of its significance.

One of the first times I tasted an alcoholic beverage was in the wine country of Switzerland, where I was having dinner with a few friends. Having grown up in the land of teetotalers, I didn't know anything about the personal or social nuances of wine consumption. The owner of the tiny, ancient restaurant where we were eating rabbit stew poured us each a glass of the best local vintage. We all clinked glasses, and I was about to guzzle my wine like Kool-Aid when one of my friends, a dapper Swiss gentleman with a handlebar moustache, stopped me.

"That's not how you drink wine," he said. "You have to keep your glass up while you look at each person in the group. I mean really *look* at them, into their eyes. Feel what they mean to you. Then, once you've really seen everyone, take a sip." The restaurant fell silent as we all followed my friend's instructions. Suddenly, the meal took on a feeling of holiness. I realized for the first time that evening how radiant my friends were to me, how precious this moment of shared time that had never existed before and would never return. As the evening passed we went from quiet, cerebral discussion to wild hilarity and back, several times. But the sacredness never faded. I've observed this ritual with all sorts of beverages ever since, even when no one knows I'm doing it. As a result I am regularly dazzled by the blessedness of feasting, whether the meal is a romantic candlelit dinner or a Coke and a bag of potato chips I'm sharing with my dog.

Some social scientists hypothesize that we modern, civilized folks have lost a great deal of psychological resonance and resiliency because we observe so few rituals. Our culture retains only a few pale relics of the celebratory rituals practiced by ancient peoples. We go to birthday parties, baby showers, maybe to church or temple on special occasions like Christmas or Easter or the High Holy Days. But we aren't a particularly ritualistic people, and I think this leaves a vacuum our nature abhors. When I was interviewing addicts, I was struck by the careful rituals that surrounded their addictive behavior, the orderly rites they followed as they prepared to take their drugs or wended their way to the casino. I noticed that it was the ritual, as much as the addictive behavior itself, that calmed them, helped drown the pain that drove every one of them. I began to suspect that they needed ritual of some kind almost as much as they thought they needed their addiction.

I've watched my own three children, who grew up with very little ritual, develop their own ways of formalizing celebration, as though the need to do this came precoded in their brains. One year, while learning the distinction between Christmas, Hanukkah, and Kwanza, the kids asked me about their own ethnic heritage. I explained that their ancestors were Celtic and Scandinavian, so we should probably observe the Winter Solstice, maybe by—I dunno—wearing Viking helmets, painting our faces blue, and eating venison. I was joking, but my children were so entranced by this idea that we actually started doing it (though we substitute steaks for wild game). This is now one of our family's most cherished yearly rituals, one that strengthens our bonds to each other by reinforcing other people's belief that we are insane.

Not all rituals are this elaborate or infrequent. My family also observes minor rites to demarcate small celebrations like watching a favorite television show. Just before one of these programs hits the airwaves, we all congregate, take the cushions off the sofas, and arrange ourselves in a specific configuration on the floor and furniture. We've never discussed this little ritual, but we all know it, and we don't vary it except under severe duress. The rites of celebration are actually more important to us, more bonding, than any television show could ever be.

You are probably accustomed to performing dozens of small rituals already, whether you realize it or not. For example, you may follow the same pattern of actions every night before you go to sleep, when you meet a certain friend for coffee, or when you exercise. In the following space, write down anything you do that typically involves a set pattern of action. Do you read the newspaper while you ride the train to work? Do you chew gum while you balance your checkbook? List anything, no matter how trivial.

CELEBRATORY RITUALS I ALREADY OBSERVE

1. _____

2. _____

3. _____

4. _____

5. _____

It doesn't matter what your rituals are. The point is simply to notice that they create a consistent behavioral "frame" that separates a certain act or situation from the rest of your life. Stop and pay attention to these rituals. You may never have thought of them before as occasions for celebration. From now on, I want you to respect each of them as a sacred rite, a passage from the workaday world into the place of feasting.

If you think you don't have any rituals at all, you're probably wrong. Read through the following section, about the content of a feast, and you will probably discover your own set of rites. If not, you'll begin creating them as you identify the centerpiece of each feast: the gift of nourishment.

Feast Step 2: Let Yourself Be Nourished

My addict friends, despite their religious devotion to the rituals of addiction, didn't benefit from whatever they used as a mood-altering device. That's because they used behaviors and substances that helped them separate from reality, so that they were lost in a kind of daze, unaware of their pain but also unavailable for pleasure, love, or real nourishment. A real feast is any activity that gives you true nourishment: love, learning, any expression of your thoughts or talents, the act of bringing your mind home to the physical anchor of your body. I'll discuss several categories of things that can count as your Joy Diet feasts, but let's start with the most obvious: food.

FEASTING ON FOOD

Yes, after reading an entire "diet" book, you have finally reached a discussion of actual food. Just because the Joy Diet is for the soul, rather than the body, doesn't mean it lacks strict rules about eating. It has two.

JOY DIET FOOD RULES (UNABRIDGED)

1. You must only eat what you really enjoy.

2. You must really enjoy everything you eat.

This means that if you really want a hot fudge sundae and you try to make do with some raw broccoli, you're totally blowing your diet. On the other hand, if you're happily porking down your hot fudge sundae and you start to feel uncomfortably full (see "blinding flash," above), the Joy Diet requires that you stop eating even if your bowl is still almost full.

I settled on these two rules as a way of normalizing my own eating, which, believe me, was no easy task. Having danced a few numbers with an eating disorder back in my youth, I've had plenty of experience with fasting, as well as my share of uncontrollable binges. When I first contemplated it, the thought of tuning in to and obeying my appetite sounded like leaving the fox in charge of the henhouse. I was sure I'd stuff myself so unstintingly that I'd end up the size of a municipal library. But after years of apprehensive experimentation, I realized that my body just wanted to establish its own normal weight and eating patterns.

Now, it is true that I went through a phase of devouring enough chocolate to cause a sharp rise in world-market cocoa shares. But this was not so much my body's real wish as a psychological reaction to having denied myself many yummy things for a long time. I solved the problem—I seriously suggest you try this—by surrounding myself with more high-quality chocolate than I could eat in twenty years.

I decided to try this method after a conversation with the checkout clerk at a gourmet chocolate shop. I'd asked him how he and the other workers kept from eating themselves into orbit. "We used to have a real problem with that," he said, "back when the employees weren't supposed to eat any of the products. But then the owners made a rule that we can have all we want. Now, every time I hire someone, I know they'll spend the first three days in the storeroom stuffing their faces. Then they'll run out of momentum and level off at about three chocolates a day. It's totally predictable. You don't stop loving chocolate when you can have all you want, you just stop wanting to eat so much of it."

I believe the reason for this is that our psychology—and also our body chemistry—tells us to hoard whatever good things seem to be in short supply. Starve yourself, and your body will urge you to binge. Then it will store every little calorie as fat, preparing itself for the next period of famine. On the other hand, if you give yourself permission to eat whatever your body truly demands, you may be surprised by how dietetically correct it wants to be. Pediatricians tell us that left to their own devices, small children—even those completely untutored by Weight Watchers—will choose a balanced, healthy diet. Adults will do the same—unless they are eating for reasons other than physical hunger.

That is a very big "unless." Please remember this: *If you are not following the rest of the Joy Diet, unrestricted eating probably won't lead to a healthy menu.* If you are unable or unwilling to sit still, face difficult truths, specify your desires, run risks, play, laugh, cry, or connect, then giving yourself permission to consume whatever you want will probably make you eat like an industrial wood chipper. On the other hand, if you're not able and willing to go on the Joy Diet, there's a high probability that you'll fail at whatever weird restrictive regimen you go on—the high-protein diet, the grapefruit diet, the all-squid-all-the-time diet, whatever. Eating is such a simple, reliable comfort that if we don't care for our souls, it's very easy to get in the habit of using food to distract ourselves from pain that has nothing to do with physical appetite.

So following the first nine steps on the Joy Diet will make it much, much easier for you to tell what your body actually wants to eat, and what it doesn't. You should feed it precisely what it asks for without blame, judgment, or stinginess. At least once a day, spend an extra buck or two on a really satisfying meal, rather than a cheaper but unsatisfying substitute. Get the high-fat version instead of the gritty, boring, pleasureless low-fat foodlike product sitting next to it. Keep asking your body—it will tell you exactly what it really prefers.

Right now, make a list of two or three things you'd enjoy eating. Don't be shy. If you just ate and nothing sounds appetizing, wait a couple of hours and try again. Remember to ask your body, not your brain, what it wants.

FEAST IDEAS: THINGS I'D LIKE TO EAT

1. _____

2. _____

3. _____

Once you've identified and located the food of the moment, it's important to eat it mindfully. That is, pay attention to the taste, the texture, the delirious pleasure of consuming exactly the food you want, at exactly the moment you want it. If you'd like, you can try a training exercise used by the pain management center at Harvard Medical School: Take a single raisin and hold it in your mouth for five full minutes. Focus your attention on the texture and taste. Notice the way the raisin changes as you push it around with your tongue, bite it, or suck on it. Many people who complete this exercise are surprised to find that they feel full afterward, as though they've eaten a whole meal. When you really experience the joy of eating, a raisin can become a feast. A whole meal eaten mindfully feels like a "feast feast feast feast feast feast."

FEASTING ON BEAUTY

One of my favorite kinds of nonedible delights is what I call a beauty-feast. We use the word *beautiful* to refer to things that please our senses of sight and sound (I have no idea why we don't usually say "That tastes beautiful," or "This is a beautiful texture," but we don't). Food, while often attractive to the eye and ear (crunch, crunch), mainly addresses our senses of taste and smell. Since we are primarily visual and auditory animals, feasting on these sorts of beauty, even with no food around, can be a glorious experience.

For example, I had a major beauty-feast right after my first book tour, a rather grueling affair that involved talking about the book I'd written until I hated talking about it the way I hate to vomit. I am obviously a person of many words, but that book tour temporarily drained my supply. By the time it was over, the thought of saying one more thing to one more person made me want to hurl myself into a live volcano. I retreated to my house with just one thought in my head: *orange*. I don't mean "orange" as in fruit, or even the word *orange*. I was just obsessed with the color. I craved orange, sought out orange things. I was entranced by the Mexican poppies outside my window, but I could also lose myself in rapt contemplation of a traffic cone or a bowl of Chee-tos. Finally, I bought a large canvas and began painting it with orange of every tone and hue. The next few days were virtually wordless. I spent them in the visual right side of my brain, while my verbal left side recharged its little batteries. It was a delicious time, one long feast for my eyes, one long rest for what little was left of my mind.

I've been similarly nourished by certain pieces—or whole genres—of music. Trying to play the piano is one of my favorite feasts, though I am what you might tactfully call inept. You may be more prone to feast your ears than your eyes, or vice versa, or you may find sights and sounds equally beautiful. What forms of beauty are your favorites? List a few below. I've given some examples to get you started.

IDEAS FOR BEAUTY FEASTS

You might feast your eyes on

1 The pearlescent paint on your new car.

2. Snowflakes falling in lamplight.

3. Your own best feature.

4. A beautifully filmed movie.

5. _____

6. _____

7. _____

Continued

8. _____

9. _____

10. _____

You might feast your ears on

1. A cat's purr.

2. A self-assembled medley of your favorite music.

3. Poetry read out loud.

4. A wind chime during a storm.

5. _____

6. _____

7. _____

8. _____

9. _____

10. _____

I'm often amazed to find that my clients, even those who can instantly name several things they find beautiful, often go years without actually feasting on these things. They own dozens of CDs and plenty of stereo equipment, but they virtually never listen to their favorite music. They know they hate the mustard color of their bathroom, but they've never gotten around to painting it their favorite shade of periwinkle blue. I often force clients—not at gunpoint, but almost—to seek out and pay attention to the things they find most beautiful. When they incorporate these things into feasts, and hold at least three every day, the world abruptly becomes much more vivid and satisfying, often breath-snatching.

You can work visual and auditory feasts into your schedule with little time or effort. Tape a beautiful greeting card to the wall of your cubicle, or turn your desk so that you can see through the window when you glance up. Play your Beethoven tapes in the car while you chauffeur the kids to polo practice or juvenile detention or wherever it is they go every afternoon. Buy the song you hear on the radio—the cheesy one that reminds you of the Love Who Got Away—and dance around your bedroom while you play it over and over. Don't just see and hear: Look and listen. These simple measures, set between the rites of celebration and thanks, will become feasts that nourish and fortify you for the rest of the day's events.

FEASTING ON REST AND RELAXATION

So far, we've covered four of the five senses: taste, smell, sight, and sound. The one remaining sense, touch, can provide the most amazing feasts yet. Leading the list of tactile feasts, of course, is good sex—need I say more? A long, luxurious massage can be added to or substituted for this kind of pleasure, depending on your state of mind, body, and social calendar. Then there are all the other spa-type activities: facials, manicures, elaborate baths, guided relaxation. Just making sure you have soft, appealing textures next to your skin can make the day feel festive. Flannel pajamas are a lovely feast for a tired hide. So are fuzzy slippers or your favorite, most comfortable T-shirt.

There's a sort of sensitivity called "proprioception" that isn't precisely touch, but seems related; it means the sense of feeling how your body is positioned. Just lying down and letting go can be a feast for the body, especially if you can get away with doing it for fifteen minutes or so right in the middle of your day. Stretching, scratching, skipping, dancing—anything that moves your body in a way that feels good can be a feast.

One more entry I'd put in this feasting category is that sublime nourishment, sleep. Most Americans get way too little sleep. Our economy loses billions of dollars every year because of accidents and illness caused by chronic sleep deprivation. I myself slept for approximately fifteen minutes between 1986 (when I started graduate school and had my first baby almost simultaneously) and 1993 (when I finally got my degree and sent my youngest child to preschool). Since then I've slept about ten hours a night. My friends have been known to address me, affectionately I am sure, as "the Sleep Slut." It is a title I relish, because I know that without the nourishment of sleep, I become a desperate, dangerous lunatic with no ability to enjoy my own existence. If your lifestyle doesn't permit you to sleep until you feel rested, start looking for ways to change it. If you have insomnia, talk to a doctor. Reclaim naps—not as the refuge of the weak and lazy, but as the birthright of every creature able to take a snooze. There may still be periods of your life when you won't be able to feast on sleep for a long time every night, but these should be kept to a minimum.

FEASTING ON BRAIN CANDY

I love television. Just love it. I always wanted my children to love it, too—parked them before the tube in their baby-swings before they were old enough to focus their little eyes. Many people are shocked when I tell them this, especially the kind of people I met during my Harvard days. Television, they exclaim, rots the mind! It is an insult to human intelligence, a

vile influence on the young, a one-way trip to terminal stupid-
ity! To all these arguments, I repeat: I love television.

The reason I'm not embarrassed to say this is because I grew
up, for the most part, in a home with no TV. Until I was thir-
teen there was nothing to do at my house but sit around reading
Shakespeare. As a result, I was able to yelp curses from the Bard
at the other children ("A pox on both your houses!") as they
pummeled me for being a complete dweeb. When someone
finally gave my family a television, I had to spend double the
usual viewing hours just catching up—thank God for reruns!
Even so, I'll never be fully culturally literate in my own country.

As a result of this background, I am acutely aware that
almost any form of brain candy is condemned when it's first
introduced to the general populace. At the turn of the twenti-
eth century, social critics warned that young people should stay
away from the cheap, imbecilic, morally questionable form of
literature known as "novels." Mozart's music was considered
altogether too catchy by many of his musical contemporaries.
Impressionist art? Shocking! Outrageous! Lewd!

The fact is that certain activities are enormously appealing
to our brains, and this upsets people who aren't used to them.
I, for one, think brain candy is not only inevitable, but gener-
ally a good thing. I believe that if Shakespeare (or Plato, or
Goethe) had owned a piece of furniture that could have shown
him unfamiliar people and distant places (even the bottom of
the ocean or the surface of another planet!) he would have
watched it all the time. Also, all these great thinkers would have
loved TV shows that made them laugh—hell, I think they
would all have *written* for television.

The same thing goes for every other type of brain candy,
from gossipy magazines to silly cartoons to weird websites. Sure,

a lot of this stuff is garbage. You can recognize the abundant dreck right away, because it's not very interesting. It doesn't feel nourishing to your brain. After watching or reading or hearing it for a little while, you'll move on, looking for something that grabs and holds your attention. More likely than not, this unusually compelling new form of brain candy will turn out to be the classic art and literature of the next century. Be one of the first to get in on the feast, boldly and without shame. If I can speak publicly about my love for scummy, half-baked news reports, unrealistic dramas, and silly situation comedies, you can, too.

FEASTING ON LOVE

In the end, there is one sort of feast that eclipses all the other kinds put together, and that is a feast of love. If you don't know what I'm talking about, keep searching until you do. There are as many different love-feasts as there are moments when one person reaches out to another, and all of them are wonderful.

To me, a feast of love is any instant (or hour, or lifetime) when human beings exchange affection. I see my fourteen-year-old son and his friends punching each other affectionately on the arm; that's a love-feast. A client tells me that something I said actually helped, and I tell him that it was his doing, not mine; that's a love-feast, too. A crowd of well-wishers shows up to cheer for the runners in a marathon, and the runners wave back. Massive love-feast. It's true that sometimes we head hopefully toward what we think will be a love-feast, serve up our hearts, and meet rejection. It's true that this hurts. But you'll find that love-feasts are so incredibly nourishing to your soul that it's worth the risk of heartbreak to attend even the smallest or most crowded one around.

Here are some ways to make sure you never miss a love-feast

you could have attended. (1) In Benjamin Franklin's words, "If you would be loved, love and be lovable." Love feasts are always potlucks: They require that each person involved brings the ability to love, somehow, some way. If you're waiting for someone else to supply 100 percent of the love you want in your life, find a therapist who's willing to accept reciprocation in the form of cash. (2) Don't keep love to yourself. If you feel it, express it—not to demand that others love you back, but simply to live outwardly the best of what you feel inwardly. The worst that can happen to your heart is not rejection by another person, but failure to act on the love you feel. (3) If you have a choice between a feast of love and any other option, go with love. As poet and love-feaster Edna St. Vincent Millay put it,

> *It well may be that in a difficult hour,*
> *Pinned down by pain and moaning for release,*
> *Or nagged by want past resolution's power,*
> *I might be driven to sell your love for peace,*
> *Or trade the memory of this night for food.*
> *It well may be. I do not think I would.*

Compared with other activities, love-feasts will mess up your life, complicate your career, wear you out, make you crazy. But I guarantee that when you look back over the time you've spent on earth, the feasts of love will be the moments and years you'll remember most joyfully, the experiences that will make you glad you have lived.

There are, of course, many types of feast I haven't begun to cover here. But I hope by now you're starting to get a good idea of what constitutes the bulk of a Joy Diet feast. Anything that feeds your true self, whether it's physical, emotional, intellectual, or spiritual, is a feast in the making. There's only one step left to completing Menu Item #10: gratitude.

Feast Step 3: Give Thanks

I think Thanksgiving was always my favorite feast because it was explicitly focused on gratitude. It's not that I'm a naturally grateful being, like Mother Teresa or Lassie. It's just that gratitude has a wonderful capacity to turn anyone's experience into the most festive sort of celebration, and I felt this as a little kid on Turkey Day. I'm not saying we should all be stupidly optimistic, filled with attitudinal saccharin designed to sweeten life's bitterness when it needs to be tasted. I'm saying that focusing on gratitude is the quickest way to determine whether or not your life really is bitter, and how to cope with it when it is. Try this: In the next sixty seconds, write down twenty things for which you are genuinely grateful. Go!

GRATITUDE STARTER LIST

1. _____

2. _____

3. _____

4. _____

5. _____

6. _____

7. _____

8. _____

9. _____

10. _____

11. _____

12. _____

13. _____

14. _____

15. _____

16. _____

17. _____

18. _____

19. _____

20. _____

If this exercise stumped you, you haven't yet become fluent in the practice of gratitude. It's not that you aren't grateful for at least twenty things—trust me, you are. It's just that you don't know it.

There's an old Sufi story about two men who encounter each other walking along a country road. One of them, a wealthy nobleman, has a bag slung over his shoulder and a dejected expression on his face. The second man, a beggar, asks him why he's so depressed. "I'm looking for happiness," says the nobleman. "I've tried everything—I've had wealth, power, position, education, lots of women, but I'm still, like, totally angst-ridden. So the other day I finally threw some stuff in a bag and set out to find myself."

"Ah," says the beggar. "I see." Then, without warning, he grabs the nobleman's bag and rushes off into the forest. He cuts through the rugged terrain until he's some distance ahead of his distraught victim. Then, when he sees the nobleman coming, he leaves the bag in the center of the road and hides behind a rock to watch.

Naturally, when the rich man sees his bag, complete with everything he was carrying when he lost it, he goes nuts with joy—jumping around, singing hallelujah, all that. The beggar, still hiding behind his rock, yells, "Strange, what it takes for some people to find happiness."

Most of us are like the nobleman, looking everywhere for happiness except in the bag of stuff we haul around every day. When I'm bored, I like to run through the preceding exercise, just saying a random, targetless "thank you" for at least twenty things I've never acknowledged before. Even when I do this several times a day, I never run out of new things for which I feel grateful. Right now, for example, I'm grateful for . . . electricity. Never done that one before. Also my very attractive new coffee mug. And coffee itself, noblest of beans. I'm grateful for the clients I saw today, for how much I enjoyed their company and admired their achievements. I'm grateful that my friend called a few hours ago and made me laugh out loud. I'm grateful for the way my daughter wears her hair (don't tell her, she'll change it), for key lime pie, for soap, for earrings, for those sticky rollers that get pet hair off your clothes. See, there you go—I'm beginning to feel pleased, even though it's very early in the morning, and I didn't have much of my usual sleep-feast last night.

A formal proclamation of gratitude always has the effect of pulling our limited attention toward things we love, and this changes everything. It's hard to worry about what you lack when you're dancing in the street, shouting hallelujahs about the stuff you've already got. In my experience, people who live this way engender far more goodwill and success than those who don't, even though they may start with less. Any feast you experience will create gratitude in you, so let it. Dwell on the good thing that has just happened. Replay the particulars again and again. Gloat. Write down the words "Thank you!" on a piece of paper, or say it out loud—to anybody who took part in your feast, to nobody in particular, to God (if you believe in God), to yourself. Create a small ritual of thanks the way you create all your other rituals, and repeat it at the end of every feast.

GRATITUDE IDEAS:

WAYS OF SAYING THANKS FOR FUN AND PROFIT

1. Buy yourself a "thank-you" treat (A gel pen! A gel pen!) to commemorate your latest feast.

2. Call a friend every time you successfully conclude a feast of any kind. Brag to each other without any modesty whatsoever.

3. Bellow like a bull.

4. Write a thank-you note and burn it, letting the smoke rise up to someplace where Mary Poppins can find it.

Continued

5. Do an end-zone victory dance, alone or in company.

6. Keep a gratitude journal, in which you write down your thanks for all your daily feasts. Oprah recommends this, and you've got to admit, it doesn't seem to be hurting her.

7. Hold a give-away, in which you reward all the people who have helped you create a feast.

4. Repeat Often

Once you've internalized all the elements of a Joy Diet feast, you can link them into a smooth, unified whole. First identify something you love, something that feeds your body, mind, or heart. It doesn't need to take long, but it must be genuinely nourishing. Then, whatever type of feast you've got planned, preface it with some small rite of celebration. Open the shutters, make the sign of the cross, take a cleansing breath, anything that works for you. Your celebratory rites may evolve from feast to feast; that's fine, as long as they help you recognize that the action you're about to take is meant to replenish you, and is therefore sacred. During your feast, allow yourself to take in all kinds of nourishment mindfully, with full enjoyment and as little resistance as possible. If guilt, anxiety, or other unpleasant habits of mind rear their nasty little heads, try banishing them by expressing gratitude for your feast, right then and there. You can start saying "thank you" whenever you like, but make sure to do it once more as a way of closing your feast.

You can manage all this very quietly, very unobtrusively, within a few minutes or across a span of hours. Just do it at least three times a day, as often as you'd eat any other type of meal.

Most people who go on the Joy Diet find they've already been feasting, but not as often as they could, and not nearly as consciously. Others discover that the life they've been waiting to live was right under their noses all along, that they've been starving while sitting at a banquet table loaded with delicacies. Derek Walcott's poem "Love After Love" describes this moment perfectly:

> *The time will come*
> *when, with elation,*
> *you will greet yourself arriving*
> *at your own door, in your own mirror,*
> *and each will smile at the other's welcome,*
>
> *and say, sit here, Eat.*
> *You will love again the stranger who was your self.*
> *Give wine. Give bread. Give back your heart*
> *to itself, to the stranger who has loved you*
> *all your life, whom you have ignored for another,*
> *who knows you by heart. . . .*
>
> *Sit. Feast on your life.*

Putting It All Together

Every menu item on the Joy Diet contributes something invaluable and delicious to the feast of your life. These aren't exotic dishes you must struggle to obtain or concoct; each is made of simple ingredients you already have within easy reach. They don't require huge sacrifices or character transplants, just a little courage and an unfaltering commitment to your own well-being. If you make even the smallest adjustments, incrementally adding each menu item to your habitual routine, your life will change in ways that will sometimes be subtle, sometimes dramatic, but always good. In the end, you'll find that you stay on the Joy Diet automatically, not because you have disciplined yourself to master some strange new process, but because you have become yourself. You were born to be open and honest and brave and playful, to laugh often, to love much, to be loved much in return. You were born for joy. Sit. Feast on your life.

MENU ITEM #10: FEASTING
MINIMUM DAILY REQUIREMENTS

1. Create a context of celebration. Observe customary, formal, or informal rites that separate a time of feasting (in other words, being nourished) from other times.

2. Let yourself be nourished. Identify experiences and substances that nourish you in a variety of different ways. Engage in them mindfully, with as much pleasure and enjoyment as possible.

3. Give thanks. This is a ritual that closes the feast, as the celebratory ritual opened it. The more concrete your means of giving thanks, the more likely you are to benefit from the experience.

4. Repeat often. It shouldn't take much effort to throw at least three small feasts for yourself every day. If possible, go for more.

CREDITS

Grateful acknowledgment is made to the following for permission to reprint previously published material.

The Acorn Press: Excerpt from *I Am That: Talks with Sri Nisargadatta Maharaj* by Nisargadatta Maharaj, translated by Maurice Frydman. (Durham, NC: The Acorn Press) 1st American ed. 1982, 11th printing 2000. Reprinted by permission of The Acorn Press.

Coleman Barks: Poem "The Guest House" in Jalalu'l-Din Rumi from *The Essential Rumi* translated by Coleman Barks with John Moyne et.al. Copyright © by Coleman Barks. Reprinted by permission of Coleman Barks.

The Edna St. Vincent Millay Society: Excerpt from the Sonnet XXX of "Fatal Interview" from *Collected Poems* by Edna St. Vincent Millay (HarperCollins). Copyright © 1931, 1958 by Edna St. Vincent Millay. All rights reserved. Reprinted by permission of Elizabeth Barnett, literary executor.

Farrar, Straus and Giroux, LLC: Excerpt from "Love After Love" from *Collected Poems 1948–1984* by Derek Walcott. Copyright © 1986 by Derek Walcott. Reprinted by permission of Farrar, Straus and Giroux, LLC.

HarperCollins Publishers Inc. and Lescher & Lescher, Ltd: Excerpt from "The temple bell stops . . ." from *The New Lifetime Reading Plan* by Clifton Fadiman and John S. Major. Copyright © 1997 by Clifton Fadiman and John S. Major. Reprinted by permission of HarperCollins Publishers, Inc. and Lescher & Lescher, Ltd.

HarperCollins Publishers Inc. and Macmillan UK: Excerpt from #11 "We join spokes together in a wheel . . ." from *Tao Te Ching* by Lao Tzu, a New English Version with Foreword and Notes by Stephen Mitchell. Translation copyright © 1988 by Stephen Mitchell. Reprinted by permission of HarperCollins Publishers Inc and Macmillan UK.

Wesleyan University Press: Excerpt from "My soul is not asleep!" from *Selected Poems* by Antonio Machado and translated by Robert Bly. Copyright © 1983. Reprinted by permission of Wesleyan University Press.

ABOUT THE AUTHOR

MARTHA BECK, PH.D., is a recovering academic who has taught sociology, studio art, and business management at Harvard and the American Graduate School of International Management. Though she is deeply committed to doing as little actual work as possible, she does periodically roust herself to act as a life coach, and in that capacity has offered advice to hundreds of individuals and groups in the U.S. and abroad. She has been a contributing editor for *Mademoiselle, Real Simple,* and *Redbook* magazines, and is presently a columnist for *O, The Oprah Magazine.* Her previous books include the bestsellers *Expecting Adam* and *Finding Your Own North Star,* and she is also the author of the upcoming memoir *Leaving the Saints: How I Lost the Mormons and Found My Faith.* Most of her useful ideas are stolen from her three children, her dog, and the Discovery Channel. You may turn to those sources or visit www.marthabeck.com for more information.